The Walking Miracle

STEPHEN RUDLOFF SR.

PAGE PUBLISHING
Conneaut Lake, PA

First originally published by Page Publishing 2022

ISBN 978-1-6624-7778-2 (pbk)
ISBN 978-1-6624-7779-9 (digital)

Printed in the United States of America

To the following people in my life who were there for me during this time of my life:

- Stephen (son) and Laura
- Edward (son) and Marisa
- Pamela (daughter)
- Kathy (sister) and Bob
- Diane (sister) and John
- Peter (brother)
- Shawn, Taylor, Jake, Eddie, Luke, Gina, and Maria (grandchildren)
- Frank and Ann, a retired police officer (personal friends)
- Lorraine and Alan (drivers)
- Linda, neighbors, and Al Salvatti a good friend

Acknowledgments

Below is a list of doctors I would like to thank for their help and professionalism during my recovery from each of my surgeries.

- Dr. Antony De Salvo (my primary doctor who saved my life at least twice as I remember) and his office staff for their help with my medical records.
- Dr. Pres Tel, my pulmonary doctor is now retired.
- Dr. Korn Beng, cardiologist, at Lankenau Hospital.

I would like to thank the doctors, nurses, and surgeons at Bryn Mawr medical specialist office:

- Dr. Mac Farlane
- Dr. Gober, skin cancer doctor
- Dr. Halpern, surgeon

I would like to thank the doctors of the neurosurgeon team who saved my life:

- Dr. Ravi Madineni, surgeon
- Dr. Abby Yochin, physician assistant
- Dr. Peter Parsells, physician assistant
- Rose Mc Devitt, office manager
- Dr. Margolies (neurologist) at Lankenau Hospital

- Dr. Scharf, surgeon at Lankenau Hospital

I would like to thank all the doctors and nurses at the following hospitals:

- Delaware County Hospital
- Fox Chase Cancer Center
- Bryn Mawr Hospital
- Lankenau Hospital
- Bryn Mawr Rehab Hospital, Malvern, Pennsylvania
- Dunwoody Rehab Newtown Square, Pennsylvania
- ICUs at the hospitals

I'd like to thank them for their kindness and understanding and also their professionalism. Thank you, and God bless all of you.

On Monday, Memorial Day, May 25, 2020, I was watching the TV. The show I was watching on the TV was a rerun from the previous year because of coronavirus. On stage were Gary Sinise, Joe Mantegna, and Sam Elliot; as I watched the entire show, these three men gave me the encouragement to write this book. I want to thank all three of you for this. God bless. The next day, I contacted my doctors to send me all my reports on my medical history for the last twenty-five years of my life. When the doctor reports started to come in, I got started to write this book. I called the book, *The Walking Miracle*.

The Beginning of my
Medical History

Starting on Saturday morning in October 1987, my customer asked me to fix her window and screen on the side of her house on the first floor. Her nephew installed her AC unit on the second-floor window the day before. As I was adjusting the first-floor window, I heard a crack. As I looked up, the AC unit on the second floor fell out. I used my right arm to block the AC unit from hitting me on the head.

Severed arm at the bicep, I fell to the ground and looked at my arm. I put a tourniquet on my arm, and then the customer came out. She saw what had happened to me, and she was terrified. I told her I was okay and drove myself to the hospital. It took twenty minutes to get to the hospital.

I got to the front doors of the hospital, and I dropped to my knees from the loss of blood. People came running out, put me on a gurney, and took me to the emergency room. Doctors and nurses came in and stabilized me. The doctors informed me that I had lost a lot of blood then they started to operate on me. They sewed 104 stitches on my arm at the right bicep area. They released me from the hospital that day. I had to return to the hospital in about seven to ten days to remove the stitches. After the doctor released me, he advised me to put vitamin E on the scar. After it healed, two weeks after, I went back to my customer's house to reinstall the AC unit properly in the window and finish adjusting the other window. The customer was sorry for what had happened to me. She paid me for the windows, and the job was completed. I was happy.

During the 1980s, I was getting headaches. I went to the primary doctor about the headaches. They put me on medication for ten days. I went back to the doctor and informed him the medicine was not working. He sent me to see a medical specialist for headaches. The doctor was a German doctor. She gave me some tests, and she informed me I had cluster headaches. The real name is Horton's cluster disease. These headaches are very painful because they affect your eyesight and cause pains in the head and face areas. When I am in my cluster stage, it could last two minutes to two hours, sometimes all day. They are ten times worse than migraines.

I now use an oxygen tank when they get really bad and last about two or three months. I am on a special diet when the cluster headaches come back. Certain foods trigger headaches.

On September 10, 1991, I was at my customer's house in South Philadelphia, two blocks away from the Melrose Diner. As I was working on the job site, the homeowner noticed brown and red moles on my left bicep. She is a nurse at the hospital in the area. She told me I should get the mole looked at. She gave me a skin cancer doctor on Broad Street; it was three blocks away. After work that day, I stopped at the doctor's office. The doctor looked at the mole on my left bicep and took a biopsy of it. He informed me to call him back in five to seven days. I called him back in five days. He informed me it was melanoma cancer. I went back to the doctor's office.

The doctor told me to lay on the table. He informed me he was going to cut and burn the mole off down to the roots. He also informed me that he might have to go down to the bone of my arm. He told me he would put me under anesthesia. I told him no, I would stay awake for the operation, and I told him to just give me a towel for my mouth to bite down on. I informed the doctor that he should not cut my left arm off since I am a general contractor and my left arm is my bread-and-butter for work.

The smell of skin and flesh was very nasty. He put a drainage tube in the wound and patched me up. He informed me to come back in seven days to check the wound. He told me to change the bandage every two to three days and don't get wet. He gave me a prescription for seven days of an antibiotic. I was lucky he informed me that I did not need chemotherapy. They caught it in time. After seven days, I went back to the doctor's office. He checked out the wound and informed me to keep the bandage on for two more weeks and to change it every two to three days. Also, to put vitamin E on the wound. The wound had to heal from the inside out. He removed the tube and gave me a clean bill of health. I did not need chemotherapy. The doctor's office is no longer there. The doctor moved to Florida.

August 10, 1997

I stopped by my mother and father's house that day around 10:00 a.m., as I normally would while working in the area. My mother was sitting in the living room on her chair when I walked in; I gave her a kiss, and she said to me to get my father in the garage, and we would have coffee. So I went outside and called my father; he was in the garage. When I walked back into the house, my mother was still sitting in her chair.

She was sweating and turning gray, and her skin was very clammy. I ran out the door and called my father, and I told him that mom was having pains in her chest. I asked my mom if she was having pains in her chest. She told me that she was going to be fine. My father came to the house and called 911. The ambulance came to the house. The MTs came and started to check my mother out. They checked all her vitals and put her on a stretcher and then in the ambulance. The MTs told my father to go with mom to the hospital, and I would close up the house and garage and call everybody. On the way to the hospital, they shocked my mother two times. My father informed me while at the hospital that they had shocked my mother one more time. After that, they put her in ICU; it took all day and night to stabilize her. I stayed with my father and my Uncle Pete in the waiting room. I left the hospital for a while to take care of a few things. I went back to the hospital to check on my mom and see if my father and uncle were okay. My father told me that there was no change in Mom. He was waiting on the doctor. I went and got coffee. We were drinking coffee when my phone rang. It was my son, Stephen; he informed me that he had laid his motorcycle down. I knew what he meant. I told my father I will be back. I met my son at the hospital in downtown Philadelphia. He was all banged up, but he was alive; to me, that's all that counted at the time. I took him home, picked up his motorcycle, and put it in my truck. I took it to a repair shop. We had coffee, then I left him and went back to the hospital.

On August 11, 1997, at 7:30 a.m., my father and I went back to the hospital to see Mom. My father went in to see his wife by himself for a while. When he came out, he informed me that Mom wanted to see me. I went to see my mom. I held her hand and told her that she was going to be fine. I told her that when she gets better, she and I would go out dancing the Irish jig at the Galway Ball in October in Germantown. She laughed and squeezed my hand. I gave her a kiss, and she said to me that she wanted to see my daughter Pamela, her granddaughter who lives in Virginia Beach. I told her I would get her there. I went outside to the waiting room and informed my father what my mother asked for he already knew. He gave me his keys to his white Cadillac; I left the hospital and left for Virginia Beach. It took me six hours to drive to Virginia Beach. I picked my daughter up; she was six months pregnant. We had coffee and started back in Philadelphia. On the way back, my daughter informed me she had to back to Virginia Beach that night because she had to be back to the navy base to report in and go to the doctor that day. I got back to the hospital, and my daughter spent forty-five minutes with my mom, and then I started back to Virginia Beach. I got her home that night and laid down for about an hour. I had a cup of coffee and a sandwich and started back to Philadelphia. I got to my father's house and lay down for about four hours, then went back to the hospital to see my mom. When I got to the hospital, my father informed me that my mom had gotten worse during the night. They put tubes down her throat and put her on a ventilator. The situation did not look good.

On August 12, 1997, my father talked to the doctors, and they told him there was nothing more they could do. The priest came in and gave her the last rites; at that time, everybody was called, and all the grandchildren came to say goodbye. All six of her children were there with my father. My mother had a living will that she did not want to be kept on a ventilator no more. I argued with my father to hold off for two weeks. But he said no because my mom did not want that. I could not face my mother in the end because I promised she was going to be fine and that we were very close. But I felt she understood how I felt. I think of my mother every day since she passed away that day. God bless, Mom.

Mom's Funeral

The funeral was done by Donahue Funeral Home. The pallbearers were her grandchildren and two sons. The eulogy was done by Mr. Bill Wright.

The Irish saying was, "May the sun warm upon your face, keep the wind behind your back, may the rain keep you alive, and may God hold your hand forever."

Mom was buried at St. Peter and Paul Cemetery in Broomall, Pennsylvania.

On January 10, 2003, I left my father's house in Havertown, Pennsylvania, to go to Clinton, Connecticut, to renovate a store for Burlington Coat Factory in the mall within the area. I checked in to the hotel in the area, then went to the store to meet the manager and set up to start the next day. I was working for three days, ten hours a day, meeting with contractors to get the job done. The weather was bad that it started to snow really bad. I went back to the hotel to get some sleep around ten o'clock when I got a call from my niece that my father was getting his last rites. I was mad that my family members had waited so long to call me. But I understand they were jealous because my father and I were very close. I went to the hotel manager and told him of my situation; I checked out, got a cup of coffee at Starbucks on the main highway, and started to go home to the hospital to see my father. It was snowing really bad. I had to stop three or four times for gas and coffee; it took me about seven or eight hours to arrive at the hospital. My father was awake. He said to me, "It took you long enough to get here." We laughed.

On January 16, 2003, my father passed away. He was the last of the seven brothers. He passed away two days after his eighty-second birthday. His close friend, Bill Wright, did the eulogy for the funeral as he did for my mother in 1997. Now all three are together again. After the funeral, I went back to Clinton, Connecticut, to finish the job for Burlington Coat Factory. While I was up there at that time, Katherine Hepburn passed away on her estate. I ate dinner at the restaurant she went to in the area. It took me six months to come to grips that my father was gone. My father and I were very close. He would want me to move on. It took a while. In 1997, my father turned seventy-five years old. And I turned fifty years old. And my son, Stephen, turned twenty-five years old. In 2022, again, if my father was alive, he would turn a hundred years old. I will be seventy-five years old, and my son, Stephen, will be fifty years old. It would be the second time in the family that it had happened. How about that?

God bless all. I miss my mother and father every day.

Cancer runs in our family. As of this year, 2022, I have had numerous colonoscopy procedures. I had a colonoscopy on August 8, 2013. I had a colonoscopy on November 18, 2016, and I had my next colonoscopy on November 2021.

On November 8, 1998, I went to see a skin cancer doctor on Copley Road, Upper Darby, Pennsylvania. I had a mole on the left side of my shoulder on my back. The doctor took a biopsy of the mole. He told me he would call me in seven days with the results. He called me in seven days and informed me it was melanoma cancer. I went to his office a few days later. He gave me local anesthesia and began to cut and burn the mole out of my back. The smell of skin and flesh was nasty. The doctor bandages me up after the surgery. He informed me not to get it wet for seven days. He gave me extra bandages to change every two days. I went back to see the doctor in ten days. He checked out the wound and informed me that I did not need chemo or radiation; he told me to keep covered for about ten more days, then I could go back to work. As of now, the doctor has sold his business, and I just found out he passed away last year.

On July 12, 2001, I went out to see a skin cancer doctor in Upper Darby on Copley Road about the mole on my back again. The doctor took a biopsy of the mole and informed me that he would call me in seven days with the results. After seven days, he informed me it was melanoma cancer again. I went to his office a few days later. He gave me local anesthesia, and I lay down on the table, and he started to cut and burn the mole out of my back. After surgery, he bandages the wound up. He informed me to come back in seven days for a follow-up. He gave me extra bandages to change the wound every two days. I had to keep the wound dry. I went back to the doctor's office in ten days. He checked out the wound. He informed me everything was good and that, again, I did not need chemo or radiation. He informed me to change the bandages every two days for another ten days; then, I could go back to work.

In November 2004, I called Dr. Miller and made an appointment to see him about the pain in my right shoulder. He checked me out and informed me to get an X-ray of my shoulder. I returned a week later, and he informed me that I had a tear in my rotator cuff; then, he set me up for an operation on December 6, 2004, in Havertown, Pennsylvania, at Wellness Center. The operation went well, and the doctor informed me that he put the arm in a sling and bandage on three areas. He informed me to change the bandages every three days for one month. He set to see me in six weeks. I was not able to work for six weeks. But I was able to drive. I went back to see Dr. Miller in six weeks. He took a look at the wounds. He informed me that everything was fine. I had to go to therapy for thirty days. Then I had to see Dr. Miller, the orthopedic surgeon. He checked me out and said to me to go back to work. He also informed me that if I have any problems with the shoulder, call right away. I was glad to get back to work after six weeks. As of 2020, Dr. Miller retired and roved out of town.

On June 15, 2011, I went to see my primary doctor; his name was Anthony De Salvo. The doctor informed me that I had to get a colonoscopy now. He told me not to come back to his office until I got the colonoscopy done. I went to Lankenau Hospital to set up the colonoscopy test on July 27. I got the colonoscopy procedure done. I had a bad reaction to the anesthesia. The doctors came into my hospital room and informed me I had malignant colon cancer resection done to the colon intestine. They put me on a soft diet for six weeks. I spent ten days in the hospital. After my release from the hospital, I had to do a follow-up with the doctors and my primary doctor in two weeks. I went back to the doctor for a follow-up. They informed me I could back to work in two weeks. Everything was fine. I did not need chemo or radiation, and I was glad about that.

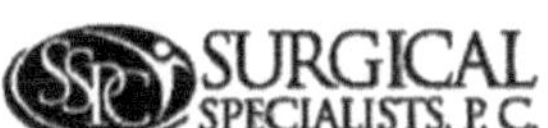

SURGICAL SPECIALISTS, P. C.

General, Bariatric, Breast, Laparoendoscopic, Gastrointestinal, Colorectal, Oncologic, Thoracic, Endocrine, Vascular, Endovascular, and Plastic & Reconstructive Surgery

Bryn Mawr Medical Building North	255 West Lancaster Avenue	915 Old Fern Hill Road
Suite 300 & 306	MOB 3, Suite 332	Building B, Suite 201
830 Old Lancaster Road	Paoli, PA 19301	West Chester, PA 19380
Bryn Mawr, PA 19010	Phone: (610) 647-3077	Phone: (610) 436-6696
Phone: (610) 527-1185	Fax: (610) 993-0668	Fax: (610) 430-6023
Fax: (610) 527-1940		

5-23-2011

Anthony Desalvo, D.O.
850 West Chester Pike, 2nd Floor
Haverfown, PA   19083

Re: Stephen Rudloff
DOB: 10/22/1947

Dear Dr. Desalvo:

I saw your patient, Stephen Rudloff, in my office on 05/23/2011.   As you know he has severe varicose veins of the right leg with multiple episodes of superficial phlebitis.   He has significant pain consisting of throbbing and aching worse towards the end of the day. He has warm an elastic support stocking for the past several years but his symptoms have progressed.

On examination he has severe varicosities of the right leg extending from the groin down to the foot with stasis changes.

He would need varicose vein surgery as the only modality to improve his situation. We discussed this in detail and he agrees to proceed as an outpatient in the Surgery Center in the near future to have this taken care of.

Thank you for referring him.

Sincerely yours,

Ronald J. Mattson, M.D.

Stephen Rudloff

On May 23, 2011, I went to see the surgical specialist in Wayne, Pennsylvania, about my right leg with symptomatic varicose veins. The doctor informed me he would operate on the leg. He explained the procedure and then gave me general anesthesia. The doctor cut the leg from the ankle to the thigh area. He installed 4-0 nylon sutures along the right leg, then wrapped the leg with sterile Kling and Elastoplast. I left the surgical center on crutches. I went back to the doctor's office in two weeks to remove all the sutures. The doctor informed me the operation healed really well. He told me to take it easy for two more weeks, then go back to work.

October 29, 2014

RE: Stephen Rudloff
DOB: 10/22/1947

Anthony Desalvo, D.O.
850 W. Chester Pike Flr 2
Havertown, PA 19083

Dear Tony,

Stephen Rudloff underwent upper endoscopy today. After informed consent was obtained, including the risks and benefits, upper endoscopy was carried out under IV conscious sedation. The patient was under continuous pulse oximetry, end tidal CO2, blood pressure and EKG monitoring. The videoendoscope was inserted under direct vision. The hypopharynx, upper, middle and lower portions of the esophagus were normal. The gastroesophageal mucosal junction was at 38 cm and the diaphragm was at 40 cm. from the incisor teeth with a small hiatal hernia present. The junction was quite irregular and multiple biopsies were obtained to rule out Barrett's esophagus. The stomach was then entered. The gastric cardia, fundus, body and antrum were normal. The pylorus, pyloric channel, duodenal bulb, second and third portions of the duodenum appeared normal. The instrument was then withdrawn into the stomach and retroflexed. No abnormalities being noted, the instrument was withdrawn. The patient tolerated the procedure well.

Impression: #1. Hiatal hernia. #2. Irregular gastroesophageal mucosal junction. Rule out Barrett's esophagus. Recommendations: Further recommendations will be made pending the results of the biopsies of which I will keep you informed. The findings of the procedure were discussed at length with the patient prior to discharge. Please do not hesitate to call if you have any questions concerning this patient. Thank you again for allowing me to participate in the care of your patient.

Sincerely yours,

Steven Nussbaum, MD.
Electronically signed

CC: Dr. Marc Surkin

On December 20, 2012, I went to see Dr. Miller, an orthopedic surgeon. I explained to him the pain in my left elbow, left hand, and fingers. He gave me a cortisone injection about two weeks later. I went back to the doctor's office and informed him that it did not help. The doctor set up surgery on my elbow and fingers on my left elbow and left hand. On January 23, 2013, at 9:30 a.m., they put me under anesthesia. After the surgery, I had a fiberglass splint on the left arm and left hand. He gave me instructions for therapy for six weeks. The doctor informed me to come back to his office to check my elbow and hand after two weeks. Then I would start therapy for six weeks and do PI on my elbow and fingers three times a week for six weeks. I went back to the doctor's office after six weeks. The doctor gave physical therapy to my elbow, hand, and fingers and released me on February 14, 2013. I was able to go back to work. I was glad to get back to work. As of 2020, Dr. Miller retired and moved out of town.

On October 16, 2014, I set up a doctor visit with Dr. Nuss Baum about my throat and lymph glands. He performed Barrett's esophagus examination; he gave me local anesthesia. The doctor informed me there was no liaison in my throat or stomach areas.

On October 15, 2019, Dr. Furman performed another Barrett's esophagus examination on my throat and lymph glands again. Everything came out normal. The doctor informed me to come in for another checkup in two years.

On October 13, 2017, I went in to see Dr. Mac Farlane, a skin cancer doctor, for a checkup. The doctor froze three pots on my face and right ear. Then she took a biopsy of my right forearm. She told me she would call me in seven days with the results. The doctor called me with the results in seven days and informed me it was squamous cell carcinoma and that it would have to be cut down to the roots. It would be called the MAS procedure. The doctor set up the procedure on November 9, 2017, with Dr. Halpern, a surgeon. They did the surgery on my right forearm and installed sutures and dressed the wound, and everything went well. He informed me to return to the office in two weeks to check out the wound. Two weeks later, I went back to see the doctor. He checked out the wound on my right forearm and informed me the wound looked very good. I did not have to come back anymore.

On March 28, I went to see Dr. Mac Farlane, a skin cancer doctor, for a checkup. She froze four spots with liquid nitrogen on my back and chest and also two spots on the left side of my head. The doctor informed me that everything was okay, and I did not need to make any appointments for six months.

On November 11, I went to see Dr. Mac Farlane, a skin cancer doctor, at her office for a complete examination of my body. The doctor found three spots on me: my right arm, forehead, and chest. She used liquid nitrogen to freeze them. Then the doctor took a biopsy of my right jaw on my face area. She informed me she would call me in seven days with the results. The doctor called me in seven days and informed me the spot on the right side of my jaw was squamous cell carcinoma, and it had to be removed by Mohs surgery. The doctor set up the date for surgery with Dr. Nalpern to due in surgery on December 12, 2019.

On December 12, 2019, I went to see Dr. Nalpern, a surgeon, at his office to have the Mohs surgery on my right jaw. He gave me local anesthesia, Lociane. He stated that he would cut and burn the area. After the surgery was over, he informed me everything went well. He installed dissoluble sutures in the wound area and informed me to keep it dry and to return to his office in two weeks for a checkup of the wound and also to change the bandages every three days for two weeks. I returned to his office two weeks later, and he informed me everything was good. The doctor told me to put vitamin E gel on the wound every two days for a month. I did not need a follow-up visit unless I had complications.

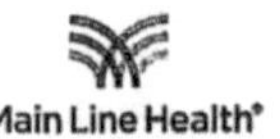

Main Line Health®

Progress Notes by Madineni, Ravichandra, MD at 8/12/2019 9:00 AM (continued)

Medications:
Current Outpatient Prescriptions

Medication	Sig	Dispense	Refill
• umeclidinium-vilanterol (ANORO ELLIPTA) 62.5-25 mcg/actuation blister with device	Inhale 1 puff daily.		

No current facility-administered medications for this visit.

Review of Systems: A 14 point review of systems was performed and aside from what is mentioned above otherwise negative.

Vital Signs:
There were no vitals filed for this visit.

Physical Exam:
Well appearing male in no acute distress.

The patient is awake, alert, oriented x 3, with fluent speech, appropriate attention span, concentration and fund of knowledge. Remote and recent memory are normal.

Cranial nerve examination reveals a left homonymous hemianopia, otherwise visual fields intact, pupils are equal round reactive to light, extra occular muscles are intact, there is no facial asymmetry and tongue protrudes midline.

On motor examination, the patient is 5/5 throughout all 4 extremities without pronator drift. There is mild dysmetria on left finger to nose testing. He demonstrates a left sided lean during ambulation with gait instability.
Sensation in intact and equal to light and sharp touch throughout all 4 extremities.

He has 2+ reflexes throughout, without Hoffman's sign or ankle clonus.

Incision: well healed without dehiscence, redness or erythema.

Data Review:
No new imaging to review during office visit.

Assessment and Plan: In summary, Stephen J Rudloff is a 71 y.o. male who is following up after 18 months from his cranioplasty on the right side. Patient continues to have residual left-sided homonymous hemianopia and right-sided neuropathic pain in the scalp. No new neurological deficits at this point of time. I recommend him to continue with exercise regimen that he is doing and also he can return to work with light duty and under direct supervision secondary to his visual field loss. All questions have been answered at this visit. I also recommend him to follow-up in 1 year time without any imaging if he is doing well neurologically. Thank you for giving opportunity to take care of Mr. Rudloff.

I, Mary Macon PA-C, am scribing for, and in the presence of, Dr. Madineni.

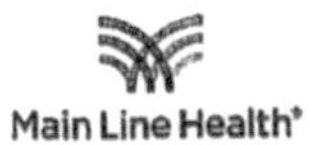

Progress Notes by Madineni, Ravichandra, MD at 8/12/2019 9:00 AM (continued)

Since last being seen the patient states he notes continued sensitivity to light, loss of left sided peripheral vision, and loss of short term memory. He continues to note intermittent numbness to the right side of his face and increased headaches during exercise and at rest. Headache is described as sharp and stabbing, located along the incision line. Headache is not the worst of his life. He additionally notes chronic left sided numbness and weakness that is unchanged. His equilibrium continues to be an issue and feels as if he is swaying back and forth. He continues to exercise three times per week and is working on weight loss.

He denies nausea, vomiting, speech difficulty, syncope, seizures, facial weakness.

Medical History: has a past medical history of Arthritis; Asthma; Cluster headaches; Colon cancer (CMS/HCC) (HCC); COPD (chronic obstructive pulmonary disease) (CMS/HCC) (HCC); Deep vein thrombosis (CMS/HCC) (HCC); Intracerebral hemorrhage (CMS/HCC); Lung cancer (CMS/HCC) (HCC); Melanoma (CMS/HCC) (HCC); Seizures (CMS/HCC) (HCC); Stomach cancer (CMS/HCC) (HCC); Stomach cancer (CMS/HCC) (HCC); Stroke (CMS/HCC) (HCC); and Vascular disease.

Surgical History: has a past surgical history that includes Colon surgery; Hernia repair; Vascular surgery; Colonoscopy; Cranioplasty; and Brain surgery (Right).

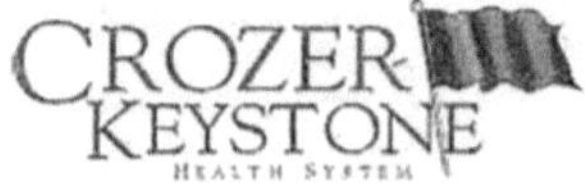

eConsultation

PATIENT: STEPHEN J RUDLOFF
ACCOUNT NO: 60011207978

PATIENT: RUDLOFF, STEPHEN J
CONSULTANT: Thomas F Prestel, Jr, MD
MED REC NO: 000-22-0643
ADMISSION DATE: 01/11/2016
CONSULT DATE: 01/11/2016
ROOM #:   CICU308 01

DICTATED, NOT AUTHENTICATED UNTIL SIGNED, OFFICIAL COPY IN MEDICAL RECORDS

REFERRING PHYSICIAN: Stacey Su, M.D.
REASON FOR CONSULTATION: COPD and lung cancer.

HISTORY OF PRESENT ILLNESS: The patient is a 68-year-old who was admitted
electively for a right upper lobe lobectomy because of adenocarcinoma of
the right upper lobe.

The patient was initially admitted to the hospital almost year ago with an
abnormality on his x-ray, which was thought to be a necrotizing infection.
He had a followup CT scan, which still showed a cavitary lesion in the
right upper lobe. However, subsequent follow up showed the lesion was much
larger and became more dense. Needle biopsy showed adenocarcinoma.

PET scan after the initial diagnosis showed intense activity in the right
upper lobe nodule, low-level activity and some mediastinal lymph nodes.

The patient was felt to be at risk for coronary artery disease. He had a
stress test, which was abnormal which required a cardiac catheterization
prior to surgery.

The patient also has a history of moderate-to-severe obstructive lung
disease. His post bronchodilator FEV1 was 54% predicted and his diffusion
capacity was approximately 50% of predicted.

The patient had a video-assisted thoracoscopic right upper lobe lobectomy
and mediastinal lymph node dissection and is seen in the recovery room
postoperatively. He is lethargic, but responsive. Heart rate and blood
pressure are all stable.

PAST MEDICAL HISTORY:

1. COPD.
2. Rheumatoid arthritis.
3. History of colon cancer treated with surgery and adjuvant treatment.

SOCIAL HISTORY: He has been a long-time smoker approximately 2 packs of
cigarettes per day for many years.

FAMILY HISTORY: Positive for coronary artery disease, also is positive for
kidney disease.

22

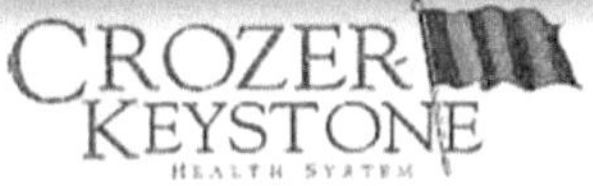

PATIENT: STEPHEN J RUDLOFF
ACCOUNT NO: 60011207978

REVIEW OF SYSTEMS: The patient is unable to give a really accurate review of systems, but does deny shortness of breath. Pain is well controlled. No nausea or vomiting. No fever.

PHYSICAL EXAMINATION:
He is a well-developed, well-nourished man, in no acute distress. Temperature is 97.3, blood pressure 106/65, heart rate 88. Exam of the head, eyes, ears, nose, throat is negative. Neck reveals no cervical lymphadenopathy. Chest is symmetrical with equal inspiratory movements bilaterally. He has good breath sounds on the left. Decreased breath sounds on the right side. Chest tube in place with a small air leak, and secretions in a small amounts in the chest tube. Heart is regular with no gallop or murmur. Abdomen is soft, nontender, normal bowel sounds. No hepatosplenomegaly. No masses. Extremities show no clubbing, cyanosis, or edema. Skin reveals no lesions or rashes. Neurologically, he is alert, moves all extremities equally.

DIAGNOSTIC STUDIES: Postoperative chest x-ray is pending.

Oxygen saturation is 98% on 2 L/minute nasal oxygen.

IMPRESSION:

1.   Adenocarcinoma of the right upper lobe, status post right upper lobe lobectomy.
2.   Chronic obstructive pulmonary disease.
3.   Rheumatoid arthritis.
4.   History of colon cancer.

RECOMMENDATIONS:

1.   We will review his chest x-ray to be sure there was complete expansion of his right lung after the lobectomy.
2.   Await pathology particularly regarding the mediastinal lymph node for staging of the cancer.
3.   Bronchodilator treatments and early ambulation.

Dictated by: Thomas F Prestel, Jr, MD
Dictated for: Thomas F Prestel, Jr, MD
Dictated: 01/11/2016
Transcribed:01/12/2016 12:10 A

23

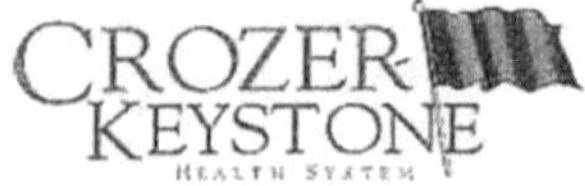

eOperative Report

PATIENT: STEPHEN J RUDLOFF
ACCOUNT NO: 60011207978

OPERATIVE REPORT

Patient: RUDLOFF, STEPHEN J
Med Rec No.:   000-22-0643
Surgeon: Stacey Su,
M.D.
Room#: CICU308 01
Admit Date: 01/11/2016
Op Date: 01/11/2016

1ST ASST:

2ND ASST:

ANESTHESIOLOGIST:

ANESTHESIA: General endotracheal anesthesia.

PREOP DIAGNOSIS:

POSTOP DIAGNOSIS:

OPERATION:

Preoperative patient identification was carried out by the attending
surgeon.

PREOPERATIVE DIAGNOSIS: Right upper lobe adenocarcinoma of the lung.

POSTOPERATIVE DIAGNOSIS: Right upper lobe adenocarcinoma of the lung.

PROCEDURE: Flexible bronchoscopy, right VATS, upper lobectomy, and
mediastinal node dissection.

ASSISTANT: Kerry Clay, P.A.-C.

PREOPERATIVE ASSESSMENT: Mr. Rudloff is a 68-year-old smoker, who
presented with an incidental right upper lobe lung nodule, which was biopsy
proven to be adenocarcinoma. The patient underwent staging, which showed
localized disease. He underwent cardiac testing, which showed him to be an
adequate surgical candidate. He was apprised of the risks, benefits,
alternatives, and agreed for us to proceed with lung resection. The
patient was taken to the operating room and placed in supine position.
General anesthesia was induced. A double-lumen endotracheal tube was
placed into the airway. Flexible bronchoscopy showed a small amount of
thick mucous secretions down all segmental bronchi. These were evacuated.
There were no endobronchial lesions. The bronchoscope was withdrawn. The
patient was turned to the left lateral decubitus position. The right chest
was sterilely prepped and draped in the usual fashion. Under single lung
ventilation, the right chest was explored. There were scant pleural

Page 1 of 2

24

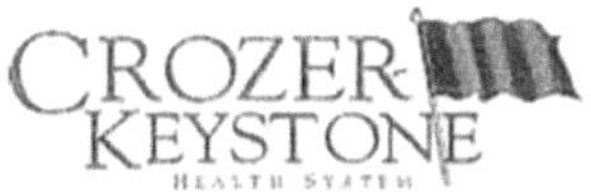

eOperative Report

PATIENT: STEPHEN J RUDLOFF
ACCOUNT NO: 60011207978

lesions that appeared to be sclerotic. One biopsy was sent for permanent
section. We proceeded with a right upper lobectomy. The hilum was
dissected. The truncus branch of the pulmonary artery was divided.
Additionally, 2 branches of the pulmonary artery were divided with an
Endo-GIA stapler. The superior pulmonary vein was divided with an Endo-GIA
stapler before the right upper lobe bronchus was divided with a stapler.
The fissure was completed with multiple loads of the Endo-GIA stapler.
Levels 10, 11, 12, as well as level 7 and 4R were sent for permanent
section. Hemostasis was achieved and Surgicel was left in the 4R nodal
basin. A 30 mL of 0.5% Marcaine was used as intercostal nerve blocks
before 28-French chest tube was directed toward the apex and secured to the
skin using 0 silk suture. The remaining incisions were closed in multiple
layers in a standard fashion. Sterile dressings were placed over the
incisions before the patient was allowed to awaken from general anesthesia.
He was taken to the recovery room in stable condition. This is an
attestation, I was present for the entire procedure.

med
Dictated by: Stacey Su, M.D.
Dictated for: Stacey Su, M.D.
Dictated: 01/12/2016
Transcribed: 01/12/2016 3:53 A
Doc#: 572791
Job#: 000793588

cc: Stacey Su, M.D.
2100 Keystone Ave
Suite 304
Drexel Hill PA 19026

Stacey Su, M.D.

Electronically Signed by SU, STACEY on 28-Jan-2016 18:01:23 -05:00

Page 2 of 2

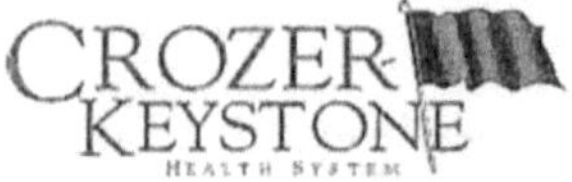

eDischarge Summary Cosignature

PATIENT: STEPHEN J RUDLOFF
ACCOUNT NO: 60011207978

SUMMARY ON DISCHARGE

Patient: RUDLOFF, STEPHEN J
Med Rec No: 000-22-0643
Attending: Stacey Su, M.D.
Admit Date: 01/11/2016
Disch Date: 01/17/2016
DOB: 10/22/1947

ADMISSION DIAGNOSIS: Right upper lobe adenocarcinoma of the lung.

DISCHARGE DIAGNOSIS: Right upper lobe adenocarcinoma of the lung.

SECONDARY DIAGNOSES: Chronic obstructive pulmonary disease, rheumatoid
arthritis, and history of colon cancer, treated with surgery and adjuvant
therapy.

PROCEDURE: Flexible bronchoscopy, right video-assisted thoracic surgery,
upper lobectomy, and mediastinal lymph node dissection.

HISTORY: Mr. Rudloff is a 68-year-old gentleman with a history of smoking,
who was found to have a right upper lobe lung nodule. He underwent biopsy
which showed this to be an adenocarcinoma. He underwent staging procedures
which showed this disease to be localized. At that point, he underwent
cardiac testing and was deemed an adequate surgical candidate by the
cardiologists. On January 11, 2016, he was admitted to DCMH where he
underwent a flexible bronchoscopy, right video-assisted thoracic surgery
with upper lobectomy and mediastinal node dissection.

POSTOPERATIVE COURSE: After adequate time in the postanesthesia care unit,
the patient was followed in the CICU Department, there he was monitored
with continuous telemetry and pulse oximetry. Vital signs were per
department protocol. He was given DVT and PUD prophylaxis throughout his
hospital course. IV antibiotics were given 24 hours postoperatively. A
Foley catheter was placed intraoperatively, was removed on postoperative
day 2 and the patient did void spontaneously without difficulty. A chest
tube that was placed in a right hemithorax intraoperatively was monitored
for the presence of air leaks as well as fluid drainage. The chest tube
was removed on postoperative day 2. On postoperative day 3, a serial chest
x-ray showed an enlarging right pneumothorax. At that time, a chest tube
was reinserted and maintained to suction and monitor. This tube was
eventually removed 48 hours after clamp trial and the subsequent chest
x-ray showed no recurrent pneumothorax at that time. The patient no longer
required CICU monitoring. He was transferred to the floor of oncology
general surgical floor. In general, the patient was out of bed and
ambulating with a thoracic walker within 6 hours upon presentation to the
CICU. He was maintained n.p.o. status and then appropriate diet was
advanced to clear liquids and to a heart-healthy diet without issue.

Page 1 of 3

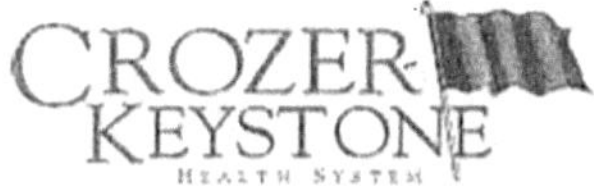

eDischarge Summary Cosignature

PATIENT: STEPHEN J RUDLOFF
ACCOUNT NO: 60011207978

Analgesia was initially maintained with the patient controlled analgesia pump while the chest tubes were in. These were discontinued. After removal of the chest tube, then the patient was maintained on Toradol, Tylenol, and oxycodone p.o. for adequate p.o. pain management. On January 17, 2016, the patient was doing very well. His vital signs were stable. He had been afebrile. He is out of bed and ambulating without difficulty. His pulse oximetry and oxygen saturation were adequate on room air at both rest and activities. He is tolerating a regular diet and had good return of bowel function and his urinary output was appropriate. At that point, he is discharged to home.

DISCHARGE INSTRUCTIONS: The patient may not drive. Diet is a heart-healthy protein enhanced diet as tolerated. He is encouraged not to lift anything greater than 10 pounds for the next 2 to 3 weeks. He may shower, but no baths, hot tubs, or swimming. He is encouraged to continue to use the incentive spirometer and green airway clearance device upon discharge to home. Ambulation is encouraged at least 2 times daily for 10 minutes and to increase as tolerated. He is encouraged to continue upper extremity range of motion exercises as instructed. He should follow up with Dr. Stacey Su in the office in 2 weeks and have a chest x-ray performed prior to that visit. He should also follow up with Cardiology as per their instruction for continued cardiac management.

DISCHARGE MEDICATIONS:

1. Oxycodone/APAP 5/325 mg 1 tablet q.6 hours p.r.n. pain.
2. Ibuprofen 400 mg q.6 hours p.r.n. mild pain and musculoskeletal discomfort.
3. He may resume his normal medications of aspirin 81 mg daily, centrum, Silver, and multivitamin as well as Anoro Ellipta 62.5/25 mcg inhaler as instructed.
4. She is also encouraged to use senna S or any over-the-counter medication to avoid constipation.

CONSULTATIONS: During this admission, the patient was seen in consultation by Dr. Kornienko of Cardiology, by Dr. Prestel of Pulmonary CICU intensivist as well as his partners, the departments of Respiratory Therapy, for which monitored his DuoNeb treatments throughout his hospital course. The departments of Physical Therapy, Occupational Therapy, and Nutrition. He is also seen by case management and social work to arrange home care upon discharge.

If Mr. Rudloff has any issues or questions including, but not limited to, fevers, chills, diaphoresis, unexplained headaches, severe mucopurulent cough, progressive shortness of breath or dizziness, any chest pain or palpitations, any persistent nausea or vomiting, abdominal pain, any calf pain or swelling, he is call Dr. Su's office immediately or report to the emergency department.

DELAWARE COUNTY MEMORIAL HOSPITAL
DEPARTMENT OF RADIOLOGY
501 N. Lansdowne Avenue
Drexel Hill, PA 19026
Phone: (610)284-8300

Thomas A. DiLiberto, D.O., Chairman

PATIENT NAME: RUDLOFF, STEPHEN J
PATIENT DOB/AGE: 10/22/1947 (68Y)
ORDER NUMBER: 90078
PT CLASS: Inpatient

MED REC #:   220643
PT PHONE: (610)505-9473
ROOM/BED: 5ONC-053101
DISCHARGED:
ACCOUNT #: 60011207978

ORDERING PROVIDER:
STACEY SU MD
2100 KEYSTONE AVE-STE 304
DREXEL HILL, PA 19026

ATTENDING PHYSICIAN:
STACEY SU MD
2100 KEYSTONE AVE-STE 304
DREXEL HILL, PA19026

ALSO SEND RESULTS TO:
ANTHONY DESALVO DO
850 W CHESTER PIKE 2ND FLOOR
HAVERTOWN, PA 19083

*****Final Report*****

EXAMINATION: **2DX CHEST 2 VIEW PA & LAT**
Date of Exam: 01/16/2016 9:00AM   **Accession #: 13394806**

IMPRESSION:
1. No appreciable change right pneumothorax.
2. Very small left pleural effusion.
3. Reactive pleural changes versus small right pleural effusion unchanged .

COMMENT: History: Right pneumothorax.

Two views of the chest were performed.

Right chest tube unchanged in position. There is very small right apical pneumothorax unchanged.

Heart size is within normal limits. No appreciable change mediastinum or hila.

Blunting of the right costophrenic angle could be due to reactive pleural changes or pleural effusion unchanged. Small left pleural effusion

No change right subcutaneous emphysema.

DEPT: 2DX
READING DR : MANJU ARORA MD
ELECTRONICALLY SIGNED BY: MANJU ARORA MD

Dictated: Jan 16 2016 10:49A
Transcribed: Jan 16 2016 10:49A
Signed: Jan 16 2016 10:49A
EDM BATCH

Printed By durj02 of 3/18/2019 11:03:58 AM -04:00

Clinical Document Architecture

Created on: January 14, 2016, 10:47:57 -0500 UTC

Patient	Stephen J Rudloff	Contact Information	117 South Eagle Road Apt 105 Havertown, PA 19083 Phone: 610-505-9473 (Home)
Date of birth	October 22, 1947	Sex	Male
Race	White	Ethnicity	Not Hispanic Or Latino
Preferred Language	eng		

Encounter	Start: January 11, 2016		
Facility/Entity	Delaware County Memorial Hospital	Contact Information	501 North Lansdowne Avenue Drexel Hill, PA 19026 Phone: 610-284-8100 (Work)
Service Location	General Surgery	Contact Information	501 North Lansdowne Avenue Drexel Hill, PA 19026
Patient IDs	Delaware County Memorial Hospital MR#: 220643 Enterprise ID: 000982333 SSN: ###-##-1421 Delaware County Memorial Hospital Patient Account: 060011207978	Document Id	2.25.308875997986026661779436003922431908514

Primary Care Physician	Anthony Desalvo	Contact Information	Phone: 610-789-5600 ext: (Work)
Admission Physician	Stacey Su	Contact Information	Phone: 610-394-4744 ext: (Work)
Attending Physician	Stacey Su	Contact Information	Phone: 610-394-4744 ext: (Work)
Consulting Physician	Thomas F Jr Prestel	Contact Information	Phone: 610-394-9860 ext: (Work)
Consulting Physician	Richard Schaaf	Contact Information	Phone: 610-259-0240 ext: (Work)
Consulting Physician	Walter Kornienko	Contact Information	Phone: 610-259-0240 ext: (Work)

Table of Contents

☑ Select/Deselect All

☑ Allergies
☑ Problem List
☑ Discharge Medications
☑ Immunizations
☑ Results
☑ Social History
☑ Chief Complaint
☑ Vital Signs
☑ Plan of Care
☑ Functional Status
☑ Discharge Instructions
☑ Encounter Diagnosis

☑ Allergies

Allergy	Category	Classification	Reaction	Severity	Onset
Dilaudid	Drug	Allergy	Unknown	Unknown	
hydromorphone	Drug	Allergy	Nausea	Mild	
No Known Food Allergies	Food				

☑ Problem List

Problem List current as of 01/14/2016

Chronic Problems							
Problem	Onset	Text	Resolved	Text	Status	Last Updated	Code
FHx Malig Melanoma		unknown			ACTV	01/11/2016	427858005
Malig Tumor of Lung		months			ACTV	12/21/2015	363358000
Rheumatoid Arthritis		unknown			ACTV	01/11/2016	69896004

Acute Problems							
Problem	Onset	Text	Resolved	Text	Status	Last Updated	Code
Chronic Obstructive Lung Disease exacerbation	12/30/2014				ACTV	01/01/2015	13645005
Community Acquired Pneumonia	12/30/2014				ACTV	01/01/2015	385093006
Coronary Arteriosclerosis	12/21/2015				ACTV	12/21/2015	53741008

☑ Discharge Medications

Discharge Medications are unavailable.

☑ Immunizations

Lung Cancer

On December 30, 2014, I was admitted to the hospital for pneumonia. I spent ten days in the hospital at that time. The pulmonary doctor, Dr. Prestel, found a lesion in my right upper lung. He informed me at the hospital before I was discharged. The lesion was small, and everything was all right. He set me up to see him in three months for some more tests at his office. Three months later, I went to see the doctor in April 2015. He gave me a lung test and informed me that I had COPD and had to put on an inhaler called Anoro. He informed me to call him for a follow-up doctor's visit in six months.

On August 2, 2016, I went to see Dr. Mac Farlane, a Bryn Mawr medical specialist, for the first time refereed by Dr. Anthony De Salvo, my primary doctor. The doctor gave me a complete checkup of my body for skin cancer. The doctor informed me I have *rosacea* on my face and nose. She gave me a prescription for *rosacea*. The doctor froze a few spots on my face, back, and arms. She took a biopsy on two spots on my body. She would get the results in seven to ten days. The doctor called me and informed me it was basal cell carcinoma. The doctor set me up to see her on November 17, 2016. At this time, the doctor gave me a checkup and topical cream for my rosacea. The doctor froze a few more spots on my arms and face at that time.

In October or November 2016, I went to see the pulmonary doctor, Dr. Prestel, for a checkup. The doctor informed me to get a biopsy of the lungs.

He called me ten days later with the results. The doctor informed me to get a biopsy of the upper right lung. The doctor called me ten days later with the results of the biopsy. At that time, he referred me to a doctor from Fox Chase Cancer Center at Delaware County Hospital. I called the doctor to set up an appointment to see her. My sister, Kate, went with me. She is a retired nurse (RN DON). The doctor informed both of us of my situation. I have second-stage lung cancer. I did not have time to get a second opinion. The doctor informed me and my sister, Kate, what had to be done. I had to get a test from a cardiologist and then get up admission tests for the operation. I got admitted to the hospital on January 11, 2016. The result of my surgery was a removal of the right upper lobe. It was malignant; it was called adenocarcinoma. I was put in the ICU section for two days. They put a tube in my right side to breathe temporarily. They transferred to a new room after two days. The doctor came in and informed me that the tube was leaking; they had to remove it for forty-eight hours. It was painful to remove. They could not give any more anesthesia at that time.

After forty-eight hours, the doctor came to my room with three nurses and reinserted the tube into my right side for forty-eight hours. After forty-eight hours were over, they came back to my room for me to check the tube was not leaking. The doctor came in the next day and told me everything was okay, and the doctor, with her nurses, removed the tube from my right side. The doctor informed me that I could now get out of bed on my own. Thank God. I was allowed to walk the hallways four times a day with a tech nurse. After that, the doctor ordered the nurses to have me get a chest X-ray every day for three days. Then the doctor came into my room to inform me I was ready to be discharged on January 17, 2016.

The doctor gave me discharge instructions. They removed the tube from my right side and installed stapes to the incisions with a sterile dressing. The doctor informed me to see her in her office in two weeks and get a chest X-ray before I came to her office. The doctor set up a registered nurse to come to my apartment three days a week to walk me in the hallways and steps and to change the bandages. After I saw the doctor after two weeks, the doctor informed me that I could go back to work three weeks later. She also told me not to lift anything more than ten pounds for two months. I was happy to get back to work with my two sons. After all this, I, again, got a break from the man upstairs. I did not need any chemo or radiation. God bless.

As of September 2020, all the doctors involved with my operation have either retired or moved on to another location from Delaware County Hospital.

On January 1, 2018, I went in to see Dr. Mac Farlane, a skin cancer doctor, for another checkup of my body. The doctor gave me a prescription for Finacea topical cream for my rosacea. The doctor froze two spots on my lower back and right side of my neck with nitrogen. The doctor thought the right side of my neck could be a cyst. She took a biopsy of my neck. The doctor would then inform me in seven days. The doctor called me seven days later and informed me that the cyst had to come out. So the doctor set me up for surgery on February 8, 2018, with Dr. Halpern to do the Mohs surgery. The surgery went well. The doctor removed the cyst on the right side of the neck below the ear. He installed fourteen sutures in the wound, seven inside dissoluble and seven on the exterior of the neck. I was to return to his office in two weeks to remove the sutures. He told me to keep the wound dry and change the bandage every three days. Two weeks later, I returned to the doctor's office; he removed the stitches and told me everything looked good and to put vitamin E gel on the wound area for about one month. I did not need chemo or radiation because of my cancer history.

On November 9, 2018, I went to see Dr. Mac Farlane, a skin cancer doctor, to get a checkup. The doctor froze three spots on my ear, elbow, and left side of my chest with liquid nitrogen. Everything else on the body was good for now.

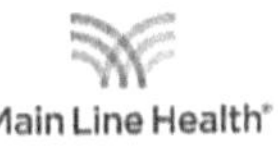

Notes

Rudloff, Stephen J
MRN: 000010734205, DOB: 10/22/1947, Sex: M
Acct #: 1100009984
Adm: 3/14/2018, D/C: 3/18/2018

Main Line Health®

Department

Name	Address	Phone
Bryn Mawr Hospital Telemetry	130 S. Bryn Mawr Avenue Bryn Mawr PA 19010	484-337-3645

Brief Op Note by Parsells, Peter, PA at 3/14/2018 8:49 AM

Author: Parsells, Peter, PA	Service: Neurosurgery	Author Type: Physician Assistant
Filed: 3/14/2018 10:38 AM	Date of Service: 3/14/2018 8:49 AM	Status: Signed
Editor: Parsells, Peter, PA (Physician Assistant)		Cosigner: Madineni, Ravichandra, MD at 3/17/2018 6:43 AM

Right Sided Cranioplasty w/ Synthetic Cranial Substitute (R) Procedure Note

Procedures:
 * Right Sided Cranioplasty w/ Synthetic Cranial Substitute

Diagnosis:
 * Acquired skull defect

Surgeon(s) and Role:
 * Ravichandra Madineni, MD - Primary

Anesthesia: General

Staff:
Circulator: Katharine Clark, RN; Stephanie Lucianetti, RN
Scrub Person: Ashley Anne Bunks, RN; Kathleen Atkinson, RN

Procedure Details
See full op note for details

Estimated Blood Loss: 150ml

Specimens:

Order Name	Source	Comment	Collection Info	Order Time
FUNGAL CULTURE / SMEAR	Bone	Pre-op diagnosis:Cranial Defect	Collected By: Ravichandra Madineni, MD	3/14/2018 9:41 AM
TISSUE CULTURE / SMEAR	Bone	Pre-op diagnosis:Cranial Defect	Collected By: Ravichandra Madineni, MD	3/14/2018 9:41 AM
TYPE AND SCREEN	Blood, Venous		Collected By: Joyce H Plank, RN	3/14/2018 6:14 AM

Drains: JP

Implants:

On July 7, 2019, I went to see Dr. Mac Farlane, a skin cancer doctor, for a checkup of my body. The doctor checked my body out and saw a few spots that needed to be frozen with liquid nitrogen on my scalp, chest, and back. She took two biopsies of two areas on my body. The doctor informed me she would call me in seven days with the results. In seven days, the doctor called me and told me that it was actinic keratosis. Everything was benign and okay. The doctor told me to see her in three months.

On December 5, 2019, I went to see my primary doctor, Dr. Anthony De Salvo. He checked out the right side of my neck, and there was a lump there. He informed me that it was a cyst beside the artery. He gave a surgeon to go see in his office. The next day, I set up an appointment with the surgeon. He checked me out on the right side of my neck. He informed me to go and get an MRI on my neck; he gave me a script for my neck. I set up the MRI test. Two days later, I called the surgeon's office to show him the results of the MRI. He informed me it was going to be tricky, but it would be fine. He set up the operation on January 23, 2020. In the meantime, the surgeon wanted me to go see my cardiologist and neurologist because I was still under the doctor's care when I had a stroke in 2017. I went to see the neurologist. He ordered me a stress test before the operation. Both doctors called the surgeon and informed him I was okay to get the operation. The operation was on January 23. They gave me local anesthesia, and the doctor informed me that the procedure went well. He stitched me up and informed me to return after ten days to remove the stitches. Ten days later, I returned to the doctor's office at Lankenau Hospital to remove the stitches. The right side of my neck healed well. He informed me to put vitamin E on the scar area. The cyst was benign; I was completely finished with the follow-up with my doctor on January 31, 2020.

On Monday, May 11, 2020, I went to see Dr. Madineni, a neurosurgeon, for my one-year checkup. The doctor was happy to see me, and he informed me that I looked good. He checked my eyes, reflexes, and arms. He also checked the lumps on the top of my head. He informed me that he wanted me to get a CT scan of my head. He was concerned about some of the lumps. I set up the CT scan a few days later, on Thursday, May 14. The doctor's office called me and informed me at 9:15 p.m. that I should get to the emergency room. I fell asleep that night, and I woke up at 7:30 a.m., Friday, May 15, 2020, and had someone drive me to the Bryn Mawr Hospital. At that time, I felt numbness all over my body and had trouble breathing. The doctors in the emergency room unit ordered an MRI, CT scan, blood work, EKG, and chest X-rays.

After about five hours, they admitted me to the hospital. They also gave me a coronavirus test; it came back negative. They also gave me a cardiogram. They put IVs in my arm. They put a heart monitor in my chest for twenty-four hours and took blood work every six hours. The doctors ordered me some medication, it was called gabapentin, all day to Saturday. The doctor came in to see how I was doing on all the tests; they all came back negative. They ruled out a seizure, heart attack, and stroke. They had me do another CT scan of the brain to check for a tumor on the right side of my head. The results came back negative. On Sunday morning, the nurse came into my room and took the heart monitor off me. They took one more EKG. As of that morning, all tests came back negative. Then the nurse came into my room and gave me another round of gabapentin. About one hour later, I had a bad reaction to the medication. The doctors came into my room and informed me they wanted me to stay in the hospital for two more days. I said no. I went home that afternoon. I stayed in bed for two days and drank water, and I had a lot of toast to flush the medication out of my system. By May 20, I felt 100 percent better. I called Dr. Madineni at his office, and he ordered another medication for two weeks to help the pain in the head from the lumps on the top head and right side of the head. As of June 10, 2020, I am okay.

On July 16, 2020, I went to see Dr. Mac Farlane, a skin cancer doctor, at her office for a complete checkup of my body. The doctor gave me a complete examination and found thirteen spots on my back, arms, face, forehead, hands, and also, the chest area. The doctor froze all the spots with liquid nitrogen. The doctor found two spots. She took a biopsy on them. She informed me that in seven days that she would call me with the results. The doctor called me in seven days and informed me everything was fine; all the spots and biopsy were benign. The doctor set me up to see her in her office on August 18, 2020, for a follow-up on three spots she froze with liquid nitrogen.

On August 12, I went to see Dr. Madineni for my one-year checkup. I had pains in my head and on the right side of my head and lumps on the right side of my head. He informed me to get a CT scan. I went to get a CT scan at Main Line Health again. My friend, Frank, took me again on Thursday at 9:00 p.m. I got a call from the doctor's assistant to go to the hospital to be checked out. I went on Friday the fourteenth of August. I was admitted that night. In the next chapter, I stayed for three days in the hospital of Bryn Mawr Hospital. As of today, I am on no drugs at all. I hope when you read this book, you'd enjoy how many medical problems I have been going through. I feel that there are others out there worse off than me. I want to help other people get through what I went through.

On August 18, I went to see Dr. Mac Farlane, a skin cancer doctor, for a follow-up visit from July 16, 2020. The doctor examined my face and arms and back areas. The results of the biopsy from the last visit were benign, and it was squamous carcinoma. The doctor froze six spots on my body with liquid nitrogen. The areas were on my face, right wrist, back area, and right leg. Everything else was good at this time. The doctor said she would like to see me in four months. I informed her that I would call the office for an appointment after the first of the year, January 2021.

My Stroke

On February 1, 2017, I woke up at 5:00 a.m. I was in my bathroom in my apartment brushing my teeth when the toothbrush fell out of my hand. I looked in the mirror and saw my face drop to my right side. Then I got this pain in my head and the right side of my head and face. I knew something was wrong. I grabbed my wallet and house keys. I looked at the door and started down the hallway toward the front doors of the apartment complex. As I was walking, the pain was getting worse. I called my friend, Frank; he told me to sit still and that he would call an ambulance for me. Frank is a retired police officer. The ambulance came and put me on a stretcher and transported me to Lankenau Hospital. On the way to the hospital, the guys in the ambulance were asking me questions; I told them my name. They kept telling me to stay with them. I don't remember anything else.

When I woke up, I was in ICU, surrounded by doctors and nurses. I don't remember too much of the first couple of days in the ICU. My sons came in and out to see me. My friend, Frank, came in to see me. The nurses checked on me every ten minutes; they put compresses on my head to get the swelling down on my head and brain. The doctors came in to inform me that I had a stroke. They called it a brain bleed. Then on February 7, at 7:00 a.m., the doctors ordered me to the operating room to take the top of my head off to relieve the pressure on my brain. The doctors put me back in the ICU in a coma. They got me stabilized after thirty days. The doctor ordered a special white helmet to wear to protect my head. Then the doctor ordered me to be transported to Bryn Mawr Rehab in Malvern, Pennsylvania, for physical therapy.

When I woke up at Bryn Mawr Rehab, my son, Stephen, was at my bedside; he had tears in his eyes. I knew something was wrong. He informed me I was paralyzed on my left side and my left eye. Then the doctors came in, and nurses talked to me. They explained to me that I would start therapy in forty-eight hours. A male nurse came to see me. His name was Reggie; he gave me a button to press any time I needed to. I was not allowed to get out of bed by myself. Reggie was a good person, and he was strict in following his orders. It was a humble time in my life because I am very independent. I had to adjust to my medical problems. I had to have a nurse dress me in the morning. I had a nurse come into my room every two days to take me to the bathroom to wash and dress me. The nurses had to teach me to brush my teeth and tie my sneakers. It took me two weeks to do these things. I was in a wheelchair for forty-five days. The nurses would take me to therapy and bring me back to my room. I had to wear the white helmet all day to protect my exposed brain.

At Bryn Mawr Rehab, I had to do physical therapy, speech therapy, and other therapy sessions, including walking balance. I lost part of my memory and part of my eyesight. It will never come back; also, I had six seizures going through all this trauma in my life; I can never drive again. I had to depend on other people to drive me while I was in Bryn Mawr Rehab. My daughter-in-law, Marisa, would bring my two young grandsons in to see me at therapy. They would say, "Pop-Pop, you can do it." It was a very humble experience after three weeks at Bryn Mawr Rehab. The doctor at rehab came in to take out the staples in my head and the drainage tub. It was very painful, but I could take the pain.

The doctor came in to see me every two days to check on me. He was a good doctor. I had visitors allowed to see me. My sister, Kate, Bob, Diane, and John came in to see me. They would stay about fifteen minutes because of my condition. To make sure I got a lot of rest. My son, Edward, would come in at nighttime to see me. We would have a lot of laughs together. After forty-five days, the doctors ordered me to go to Dunwoody Rehab in Newtown Square, Pennsylvania, for forty-five days. One night, my son, Edward, came to see me at Bryn Mawr Rehab, and he gave me some blood oranges. I ate two oranges that night; they were very good, and it tasted like eating sugar. I guess the medication I was on at that time covered me to have a seizure. The next day, they took me by ambulance to Paoli Hospital for tests the whole day. They took me back to Bryn Mawr Rehab that night; I lost two days of therapy. As of today, I never had another blood orange again. The doctors came into my room and informed me that I was going to be transferred to Dunwoody Rehab in three days. So my son, Edward, informed me that he got permission to have a pizza party downstairs for me. My daughter-in-law, Marisa, came in with my two grandsons, Eddie and Luke. My sister, Diane, John, and my daughter, Pamela, came to the party. We all had a good time. The next day, my good friend, Al Saluatti, came in to see me. We had some laughs; it was good to see him.

On March 27, 2017, I went to see Dr. Madineni for a follow-up as requested by the doctor, who kept in touch with my son, Stephen, by texting each other. My friend, Frank, took me this day to see the doctor. He gave me a complete checkup and ordered me to get an MRI on my head. I had the MRI at Main Line Health, and I gave the disc to the doctor. The doctor texted my son, Stephen, and told my son everything was good at that time. Dr. Madineni texted my son, Stephen, that he would like to see me in six weeks. Time to set up the operation to put the top of my head back on.

Dr. Madineni texted my son, Stephen, around May 15, 2017, for me to get an MRI at Main Line Health. My friend, Frank, took me to get the MRI. The doctor got the results of the MRI and texted my son to set up the operation on May 31, 2017, at Lankenau Hospital to put the top of my head back on. It was Memorial Day weekend. The operation was on Friday. The doctor informed my son that it would take three to four hours for the operation. When I woke up, I was placed in ICU for five days. Dr. Abby Yochin, Dr. Madineni's assistant, came into the ICU and removed the drainage tube from the back of my head. The doctor bandaged the top of my head and informed me that I would be transferred to a private room on the second floor for five days. I had to do some therapy and was allowed out of bed on my own. I was discharged to go home after five days. The doctor got me up to see Dr. Madineni for a follow-up in June. The doctor informed me that everything went well. I went home to rest for a couple of weeks. On June 19, 2017, I went to see Dr. Madineni for a follow-up and complete checkup of my head and body. The doctor removed the staples in my head. The doctor informed me and my son, Stephen, that everything looked good. The doctor told me and my son that he'd see me in five or six months for a checkup.

On Monday, I met with the therapy nurses who were to take care of me while I was in Dunwoody Rehab. I was informed that I would be here for a least forty-five days. Then I would be able to go home to my apartment. After three weeks of therapy at Dunwoody Rehab, the doctors informed me and my sons that they could not do any more for me. At that time, my therapy was completed. My son, Stephen, came in to pick me up and take me to my apartment with the white helmet on to protect my brain. It felt good to get home to my apartment and sleep in my own bed. My first night at home was tough on me. I thanked the man upstairs for not taking me home at this time.

On April 15, 2017, I was transported by ambulance to Dunwoody Rehab in Newtown Square, Pennsylvania. I checked in on Friday afternoon. I was met by a male nurse. He helped me into my room. I unpacked my clothes, and he informed me that dinner would be at 5:00 p.m. The nurses came into my room to check me out and ask questions and check my vitals at that time. I was not allowed any visitors that weekend. They put me back on oxygen. I was allowed to take a shower by myself for the first time. I was happy to be able to do things for myself. I also was allowed to walk the hallways; I was not allowed to leave the second floor by myself.

For the next two weeks, I sat in my apartment and watched TV and rested my body. I had to wear my helmet all the time. I would go anywhere outside my apartment. It took me two weeks to go outside by myself. I would walk around the apartment building to get fresh air. My sons, Stephen and Edward, would call me if the helmet was on and to see if I needed anything at that time. I had to go to the doctor for a follow-up. My son, Stephen, would take me to doctor visits when possible. My friend, Frank, would take me to the doctor. Also, when my son, Stephen, could not take me.

On November 30, 2017, I went to see Dr. Madineni for a follow-up appointment to give me a complete physical on my head, eyes, balance, and reflexes. My son, Stephen, was there with me. The doctor informed both of us that everything was good. He also informed me about cutting back on the medication I was taking at this time.

The Second Time They Removed the Top of My Head

On January 15, 2018, I went to see Dr. Madineni about pains in my head and body. He checked me out and informed me to get a CT scan of my head by Main Line Health. My friend, Frank, took me to the doctor on that day, and he took me on January 16 to get a CT scan on my head at Main Line Health in Broomall, Pennsylvania. On January 22, 2018, my son and I went to see Dr. Madineni with the results of the CT scan. The doctor informed me and my son, Stephen, that the head cap on my head was deteriorating and had to be removed because there was no blood flow going into the cap. The doctor had me and my son go see the specialist about measuring my head with a new synthetic cranial substitute for my head. We were told it would take three weeks to get this. The doctor ordered a prescription to lessen the pain in my head. Dr. Madineni texted my son, Stephen, and set up the surgery on my head in February 2018 at Bryn Mawr Hospital. The operation went well at that time, and I spent days in the hospital, three days in ICU, and seven days in a private room. I had to do five days of therapy. The doctor came in to inform me I was going to be discharged in a couple of days. I stayed on medication for a couple of months. Until I went back to see Dr. Madineni for a follow-up appointment in March 2018.

On March 18, 2018, I went to see Dr. Madineni for a checkup. The doctor informed me and my son, Stephen, that everything was going well. He informed me I was going to stay on the medication for now. He informed me and my son that he would like to see me in three months. In June 2018, I went to see Dr. Madineni for a follow-up meeting. He checked me up on my head and reflexes. He informed me and my son, Stephen, that everything was very good. At that time, the doctor informed me that he would cut back on my medication for about sixty days.

On August 14, I went to see Dr. Madineni at his office for a checkup. My friend, Frank, took me that day. The doctor checked me out really well that day and informed me that I did not have to take any more medications; I was happy then. I do not like to take drugs. I have a high tolerance for pain. The doctor informed me that he would like to see me in one year for a checkup. I told him I would call for an appointment in one year.

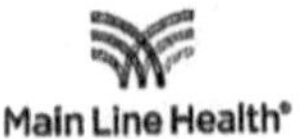
Main Line Health®

Progress Notes by Madineni, Ravichandra, MD at 9/10/2018 9:30 AM (continued)

History of Present Illness:
Stephen J Rudloff is a 70 y.o. who presents today for routine post operative follow up. The patient underwent a right sided cranioplasty on 3/14/2018. The patient initially presented with a right sided intraparenchymal hemorrhage for which he underwent a craniectomy in February of 2017, followed by cranioplasty in June of the same year. The patient subsequently had reabsorption of his bone flap which prompted his most recent cranioplasty. Since last being seen the patient states he has intermittent sensitivity to light, swelling/flushing into the right side of his face, associated with intermittent numbness in the same area and a feeling "like fluid running down". Otherwise he is without complaint. No headaches, nausea, vomiting or weakness.

Medical History: has a past medical history of Arthritis; Asthma; Cluster headaches; Colon cancer (CMS/HCC) (HCC); COPD (chronic obstructive pulmonary disease) (CMS/HCC) (HCC); Deep vein thrombosis (CMS/HCC) (HCC); Intracerebral hemorrhage (CMS/HCC) (HCC); Lung cancer (CMS/HCC) (HCC); Melanoma (CMS/HCC) (HCC); Seizures (CMS/HCC) (HCC); Stomach cancer (CMS/HCC) (HCC); Stomach cancer (CMS/HCC) (HCC); and Stroke (CMS/HCC) (HCC).

Surgical History: has a past surgical history that includes Colon surgery; Hernia repair; Vascular surgery; Colonoscopy; Cranioplasty; and Brain surgery (Right).

Family History: family history is not on file.

Social History:
Social History

Social History
- Marital status: Single
  Spouse name: N/A
- Number of children: N/A
- Years of education: N/A

Social History Main Topics
- Smoking status: Former Smoker
  Types: Cigarettes
  Quit date: 2016
- Smokeless tobacco: Never Used
- Alcohol use   Yes
  Comment: hasnt had liquor in 4 months
- Drug use: No
- Sexual activity: Defer

Other Topics   Concern
- None

Social History Narrative
- None

Allergies: No Known Allergies

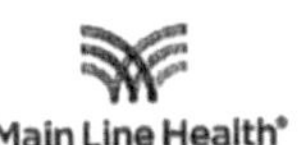

Main Line Health®

Progress Notes by Madineni, Ravichandra, MD at 9/10/2018 9:30 AM (continued)

Assessment and Plan: In summary, Stephen J Rudloff is a 70 y.o. male who is 6 months postop from a redo right-sided cranioplasty with a synthetic bone flap presenting with complaints of having numbness in the scalp and right side of the face as well as difficulty with vision which are secondary to having some neuropathy as well as a left homonymous hemianopia from a right-sided parietal occipital ICH. I explained to the patient about the imaging findings and the nature of brain injury he had secondary to ICH and that these deficits are probably permanent and he may have these symptoms for the rest of his life which he needs to overcome and managed to adjust his lifestyle accordingly. Patient would like to know if he can drive and I have counseled him many times that he cannot drive with the existing homonymous hemianopia. Patient is accompanied by his son at this visit and they understand the above. I will see him back in about 1 year time. Thank you for giving opportunity to take care of Mr. Rudloff.

I, Peter Parsells PA-C, am scribing for, and in the presence of, Dr. Madineni.

I, Dr. Ravi Chandra Madineni, personally performed the services described in this documentation as scribed by Peter Parsells PA-C in my presence, and it is accurate and complete

Electronically signed by Madineni, Ravichandra, MD at 9/29/2018 12:24 PM

Department

Name	Address	Phone	Fax
Main Line Health Jefferson Neurosurgery at Bryn Mawr Hospital	830 Old Lancaster Road MOB North Suite 209 Bryn Mawr PA 19010	610-525-1061	610-525-3509

Progress Notes by Madineni, Ravichandra, MD at 8/12/2019 9:00 AM

Author: Madineni, Ravichandra, MD	Service: —	Author Type: Physician
Filed: 8/17/2019 8:25 AM	Encounter Date: 8/12/2019	Status: Signed
Editor: Madineni, Ravichandra, MD (Physician)		

08/12/19

Re: Stephen J Rudloff
DOB: 10/22/1947

Chief Complaint:
Follow up

History of Present Illness:
Stephen J Rudloff is a 71 y.o. left handed male who presents for 1 year follow up.

The patient underwent a right sided cranioplasty on 3/14/2018. The patient initially presented with a right sided intraparenchymal hemorrhage for which he underwent a craniectomy in February of 2017, followed by cranioplasty in June of the same year. The patient subsequently had reabsorption of his bone flap which prompted his most recent cranioplasty.

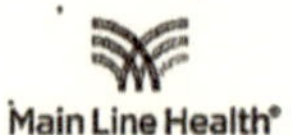

Comparison: Multiple prior studies, most recent CT brain dated 2/15/2017.
Technique: Multiplanar MR imaging of the brain was performed before and
after administration of intravenous contrast (8) mL of Gadavist).
Findings:
Status post right temporoparietal craniectomy with protrusion of the
right frontal, parietal and occipital lobes through the craniectomy
defect. Subacute lobar parenchymal hemorrhage within the right parietal
and occipital lobes measures 4.5 x 1.9 x 3.1 cm and has contracted when
compared to prior study.   There is ex-vacuo dilation of the right
lateral ventricle. Presence of T1 hyperintensity within the hemorrhage
limits evaluation on the post contrast images. Faint enhancement is seen
at the periphery of the hemorrhage, but no definite tumor-like
enhancement noted. No enhancement noted in these regions on the prior
MRI, suggesting that these areas are most likely reactive. Small vessel
disease is stable. Cerebellar tonsils are in normal location. The sella
appears unremarkable. The major intracranial flow voids at the skull base
are normal in appearance. Increased signal within the right mastoid air
cells.
IMPRESSION:
Expected further evolution of subacute lobar parenchymal hemorrhage
within the right parieto-occipital lobe. Decreased regional mass effect
and decreased protrusion of the brain through the craniectomy defect.
I certify that I have reviewed this examination and agree with this
report.
Michael Ferrell, MD
Transcribed by: n/a :Apr 3 2017 4:06P
Dictated by: CRISTINA J QUINTERO :Apr 3 2017 3:08P
Dictation signed by:MICHAEL S FERRELL MD:Apr 3 2017 4:29P
CPT Code:

Testing Performed By

Lab - Abbreviation	Name	Director	Address	Valid Date Range
68 - Unknown	SOARIAN HISTORICAL CONVERSION	Unknown	Unknown	03/08/17 1419 - Present

CT HEAD WITHOUT IV CONTRAST [17401116]

Electronically signed by: **Interface, Radiology Results Conversion on 08/17/17 0000** Status: **Completed**
Ordering user: Interface, Radiology Results Conversion 08/17/17   Ordering provider: Madineni, Ravichandra, MD 0000
Authorized by: Madineni, Ravichandra, MD

CT HEAD WITHOUT IV CONTRAST [17401116] Result status: Final result

Ordering provider: Madineni, Ravichandra, MD 08/17/17 0000   Resulted by: Provider, Historical, MD
Accession number: 13130415 Resulting lab: SOARIAN HISTORICAL CONVERSION
Narrative:
CAT SCAN - Aug 17 2017 8:30AM - CT BRAIN WITHOUT CONTRAST
CLINICAL HISTORY: I 61.1. Right cerebral hemorrhage.
COMMENT:
An unenhanced CT scan of the brain was performed from the foramen magnum
to the vertex. Coronal and sagittal reconstructions were obtained.
CT DOSE: One or more dose reduction techniques (e.g. automated exposure
control, adjustment of the mA and/or kV according to patient size, use of
iterative reconstruction technique) utilized for this examination.
Comparison: Several priors, the most recent of which was performed
6/5/2017.
Findings:
The study is degraded by artifact from patient motion. Postsurgical

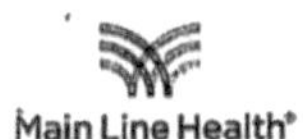

<table>
<tr><td></td><td>Orders/Results</td><td>Rudloff, Stephen J
MRN: 000010734205, DOB: 10/22/1947, Sex: M
Acct #: 2003271280
Adm: 2/15/2017, D/C: 2/15/2017</td></tr>
</table>

changes are present from a right-sided craniotomy. The previously seen
surgical skin staples have been removed. There is a significant interval
decrease in the size of the previously seen fluid collection subjacent to
the craniotomy site. Dural thickening/residual collection is present in
this region measuring up to 2 mm. Previously, an 8 mm collection was
present in this region. Right-sided occipitoparietal and posterior
temporal encephalomalacia appears stable. There is associated ex vacuo
dilatation of the atrium and occipital horn of the right lateral
ventricle. Patchy white matter hypoattenuation is present which is
nonspecific but likely represents chronic microvascular ischemic changes.
There is no gross new loss of the gray-white matter discrimination to
suggest an acute large vascular territorial infarct. No new acute
intracranial hemorrhage is identified. The ventricles are midline and the
basilar cisterns are patent.
Ethmoid air cell mucosal thickening is present. The remainder of the
visualized portions of the paranasal sinuses and the mastoid air cells
appear patent.
IMPRESSION:
Motion degraded study.
Postoperative changes with significant interval decrease in the size of
the previously seen fluid collection subjacent to the craniotomy, now
measuring up to 2 mm in maximal thickness, as above.
Stable right-sided occipitoparietal and posterior temporal
encephalomalacia.
Other stable chronic and incidental findings, as above.
Transcribed by: n/a :Aug 17 2017 11:31A
Dictated by: JENIFER SLONE :Aug 17 2017 11:24A
Dictation signed by:JENIFER SLONE :Aug 17 2017 11:32A
CPT Code: 70450

Testing Performed By

Lab - Abbreviation	Name	Director	Address	Valid Date Range
68 - Unknown	SOARIAN HISTORICAL CONVERSION	Unknown	Unknown	03/08/17 1419 - Present

X-RAY CHEST 2 VIEWS [31948342]

Electronically signed by: **Jones, Pamela R on 03/09/18 0910**	Status: **Completed**

This order may be acted on in another encounter.
Ordering user: Jones, Pamela R 03/09/18 0910   Authorized by: Madineni, Ravichandra, MD
Indications of use: Pre-op major surgery
Diagnoses
Zygomatic hyperplasia [M95.2]
Preop examination [Z01.818]

X-RAY CHEST 2 VIEWS [31948342]	Resulted: 03/09/18 1135, Result status: Final result

Resulted by: Performed: 03/09/18 1036 - 03/09/18 1040
Stassi, John, MD
Damle, Rohan N, MD
Accession number: 1000025522   Resulting lab: FOUNDATION RADIOLOGY SYSTEM
Narrative:
CLINICAL HISTORY: Preoperative evaluation of the chest..

COMMENT: Erect PA and lateral views of the chest were obtained.

COMPARISON: Chest CT from 10/31/2017 and chest radiograph from 2/8/2017

The lungs are hyperinflated. There is no focal consolidation, pneumothorax, eOperative and Procedure Report - 2/7/2017 - 1 pg(s)

MAIN LINE HOSPITALS

Lankenau Hospital

OPERATIVE REPORT

Patient Name:	RUDLOFF,STEPHEN
MR#:	765629
Visit #:	4005045106
DOB:	10/22/1947
Admit Date:	01/31/2017
Procedure Date:	02/07/2017

PREOPERATIVE DIAGNOSIS:
Right-sided parietooccipital intracerebral hemorrhage and brain herniation.

POSTOPERATIVE DIAGNOSIS:
Right-sided parietooccipital intracerebral hemorrhage and brain herniation.

PROCEDURE PERFORMED:
Right-sided frontotemporoparietal craniectomy, decompression and evacuation of hematoma.

SURGEON:
Ravichandra Madineni, MD, attending.

ASSISTANT:
Lisa Black, PA.

ANESTHESIA TYPE:
General endotracheal anesthesia.

ESTIMATED BLOOD LOSS:
300 mL.

COMPLICATIONS:
None.

FEBURARY 1ST 2017

PATHOLOGY:
Sent for final.

FEB 1ST

CLINICAL HISTORY:
Mr. Rudloff is a 69-year-old gentleman who was admitted on ~~2/~~2017 with the sudden onset of headache and found to have a right-sided occipital intracerebral hemorrhage and was admitted to Lankenau Hospital and kept in the ICU for observation. The patient, over a period of time, gradually shown on the CT scan of head, had worsening of the hematoma with expansion and increase in size causing mass effect with edema and some herniation. On 02/07/2017 morning, the patient complained of worsening of his headaches with nausea and multiple episodes of vomiting and was found to have, on the CT scan, worsening of her ICH as well as surrounding edema and herniation with the midline shift of 10 mm. The patient was emergently taken to the OR, after thoroughly discussing with the family all the possible treatment options and surgical complications were explained.

DESCRIPTION OF PROCEDURE:
The patient was brought to the OR, and general endotracheal anesthesia was performed by the department of anesthesia. The patient was supine on the operating room table with a shoulder bump, and the head was turned towards the left. Prior to intubation, the patient had got 75 mL of Mannitol, 2 grams of Ancef as a preoperative antibiotic, and intermittent compression devices were applied to both the legs. The patient's head was fixed in a

Page 1 of 2

. Page 1 of 2 - Printed By:CUSTOM10\JOKF_stm_server On:5/29/2018 3:52:12 PM -04:00

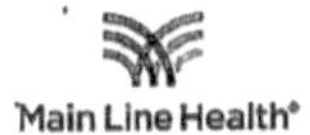

Rudloff, Stephen J
MRN: 000010734205, DOB: 10/22/1947, Sex: M
Acct #: 4005045106
Adm: 1/31/2017, D/C: 2/13/2017

eOperative and Procedure Report - 2/7/2017 - 1 pg(s)

MAIN LINE HOSPITALS

Lankenau Hospital

OPERATIVE REPORT

Patient Name: RUDLOFF,STEPHEN
MR#:   765629

Mayfield 3-pin frame. Once the patient was under anesthesia, the hair was clipped, and head was prepped using Betadine scrub and Betadine solution. Once the prep was dry, the sterile area was draped with towels and a sterile drape. So, a skin incision was performed using a #10 blade, and the scalp flap was elevated, including the temporalis muscle. Once the skull was adequately exposed, burr holes were performed using Midas Rex perforator. And, after releasing the underlying dura, next, craniotomy was performed using the foot plate of the Midas Rex drill, and a large frontotemporoparietal craniotomy was performed. Bone flap was elevated after releasing the dura. Thorough hemostasis was achieved as this surgery was being progressed. The dura was opened in a cruciate fashion with multiple leaflets. The brain was under tension. Surface of the brain had evidence of underlying hematoma. A small area of corticectomy was performed, and the hematoma was partially evacuated. No active arterial bleeders were noted. Blood clot was sent for pathology. Hemostasis was achieved using the electrocautery bipolar, Surgicel, and FloSeal. Hematoma cavity was copiously irrigated with saline irrigation. After achieving thorough hemostasis, dural leaflets were placed back loosely, and the dural defect was covered with a DuraGen graft. A 7-French flat JP drain was placed and tunneled out through a separate stab incision in the scalp. Next, 2-0 interrupted Vicryl sutures were used to close the galeal layer. Staples were used to close the scalp. Sterile dressing was applied. The patient was transported in stable condition to CT scan and then to neuro ICU, intubated. During the surgery, antibiotic dose was redosed.

I was present for all the critical portions of this procedure as well as available at all times immediately.

Ravichandra Madineni, MD

Dictated by:

DD: 02/09/2017 00:00:00
DT: 02/09/2017 15:35:27
TransID:7542006/Dict Job #: 0
iChart Voice #: 0/iChart Text #: 56494770

CC: Ravichandra Madineni, MD.

Edited By Madineni, Ravichandra 10-Feb-2017 09:03:21 -05:00

Signed by Madineni, Ravichandra on 10-Feb-2017 09:03:21 -05:00

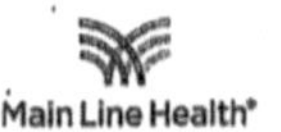

Main Line Health®

MARCH.

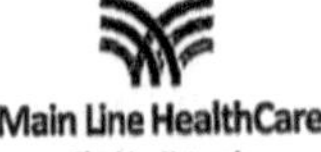

Main Line HealthCare
Physician Network

Main Line Healthcare Neurosurgery

Tel 610.525.1061
Fax 610.525.3509
mainlinehealth.org/mlhc

830 Old Lancaster Road
Medical Office Building North, Suite 209
Bryn Mawr, PA 19010

March 27, 2017

Anthony J. DeSalvo, D.O.
850 West Chester Pike
Suite 201
Havertown, PA 19083

Re: STEPHEN J RUDLOFF
DOB: 10/22/1947

Dear Dr. DeSalvo:

CHIEF COMPLAINT: Status post right-sided craniectomy for intracerebral hemorrhage.

HISTORY OF PRESENT ILLNESS: Mr. Rudloff is here for a seven-week followup from having right-sided hemicraniectomy and decompression for intracranial hemorrhage on February 7, 2017 at Lankenau Hospital. The patient was subsequently discharged to rehab, and then he was discharged from rehab to home. The patient says he is overall feeling much better. He has recovered from his left-sided hemiparesis; however, he still has visual field cut with left homonymous hemianopsia. The patient says he does have some pain and dysesthesias along the scalp incision, especially the posterior part. No history of any headache. No nausea or vomiting. No history of diplopia. No history of weakness of extremities. No history of any seizures.

PAST MEDICAL HISTORY: Significant for lung cancer and colon cancer.

PAST SURGICAL HISTORY: Right-sided hemicraniectomy February 7, 2017, colon cancer surgery February 10, 2014, and lung cancer surgery January 9, 2016.

ALLERGIES: No known drug allergies.

MEDICATIONS: Keppra 500 mg twice a day.

FAMILY HISTORY: Significant for heart attack in both parents, who are deceased.

SOCIAL HISTORY: He quit smoking on January 2, 2017, but however has previously forty years of smoking. He denies any alcohol or illicit drugs.

PHYSICAL EXAMINATION: Vital signs are reviewed, and documented in the chart. General appearance, Mr. Rudloff is a very pleasant, 69-year-old gentleman who stands 6 feet 1 inch tall, and weighs about 183 pounds. He is well built and nourished. Appears of stated age. Head normocephalic. Right-sided craniectomy defect. Pupils bilaterally equal and reactive. Extraocular movements intact. He has a left-sided homonymous hemianopsia. Neck is soft, supple. No JVD, no bruits. Cardiovascular system, S1, S2 is heard. Regular rate and rhythm. Respiratory system, normal breath sounds heard. Extremities, no cyanosis, clubbing, or edema. Pulses 2+.

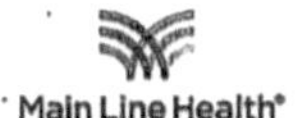

Main Line Health®

RUDLOFF, STEPHEN J
March 27, 2017
Page 2

NEUROLOGICAL EXAMINATION: The patient is awake, alert, oriented x3. He is following commands. He has a normal attention span and concentration. Recent and remote memory is intact. He has normal speech without any dysphagia. Pupils are equal, round, and reactive to light. Extraocular movements are intact. V1 through V3 sensations are normal. Face is symmetric, and normal in strength. Lower cranial nerves normal. Uvula and palate elevate normally. Can hear finger rub in both ears. Shoulder shrug is normal. Tongue is midline. Motor exam, muscle tone in both normal. Strength 5/5 in all extremities in all muscle groups. No pronator drift. Sensations normal to light touch and pinprick. Deep tendon reflexes 2+. Negative for Hoffman's and Babinski's. Normal antalgic gait. No dysmetria on finger-to-nose test.

DATA REVIEW: Currently, there are no radiological examinations to review.

ASSESSMENT/PLAN: Mr. Rudloff is seven weeks from having a right-sided craniectomy for her decompression of intracerebral hemorrhage. He is neurologically doing much better, and he has recovered from his left hemiparesis almost completely. His strength is normal. He, however, has residual left-sided homonymous hemianopsia. The patient is accompanied by his son for this visit, and we discussed about further course of management. I would like to see him back with MRI of the brain with and without gadolinium to rule out any underlying tumor. I gave a script for the MRI of the brain. I also recommended they can call me when the MRI is done so I can take a look. We will plan to put back the bone flap in the next four to six weeks or after the MRI is done. I answered all their questions, and we agree with the plan. They can call me with any questions at this point.

Sincerely,

ELECTRONICALLY SIGNED BY Ravi Chandra Madineni, MD ON 04/06/2017 09:45
Ravi Chandra Madineni, MD

cc: Anthony J. DeSalvo, D.O., 850 West Chester Pike, Suite 201, Havertown, PA 19083,
FAX: 610-789-7836

59

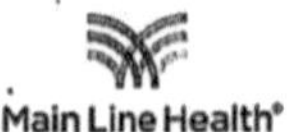

Media Scans

Rudloff, Stephen J
MRN: 000010734205, DOB: 10/22/1947, Sex: M
Acct #: 4005165680
Adm: 5/31/2017, D/C: 6/6/2017

eOperative and Procedure Report - 5/31/2017 - 1 pg(s)

MAIN LINE HOSPITALS

Lankenau Hospital

OPERATIVE REPORT

Patient Name:	RUDLOFF,STEPHEN
MR#:	765629
Visit #:	4005165680
DOB:	10/22/1947
Admit Date:	05/31/2017
Procedure Date:	05/31/2017

PREOPERATIVE DIAGNOSIS: Right-sided frontotemporoparietal cranial defect.

POSTOPERATIVE DIAGNOSIS: Right-sided frontotemporoparietal cranial defect.

PROCEDURE: Right-sided frontotemporoparietal cranioplasty with autologous bone flap more than 5 cm.

SURGEON: Ravichandra Madineni, MD

ASSISTANT: Peter Parsells, PA

ANESTHESIA: General endotracheal.

SPECIMENS: Nil.

COMPLICATIONS: None.

One 10-French flat JP drain.

INDICATION FOR PROCEDURE: Mr. Rudloff is a 69-year-old gentleman who had right-sided intracerebral hemorrhage in February 2017 and subsequently underwent a right-sided frontotemporoparietal decompressive hemicraniectomy on 02/07/2017 from which he recovered and was subsequently discharged to rehabilitation. The patient was followed up in clinic and had CT scan of the head as well as MRI of the brain and was ruled out to have any underlying pathology. The patient is planned for a right-sided cranioplasty with autologous bone flap of more than 5 cm and I discussed the procedure and as well as the complications in detail with the patient and his son, who were present at office visit. Complications included, but not limited to, infection, bleeding, paralysis, seizures, stroke, weakness of the left side of the body, sensory dysfunction, CSF leak, need for further procedure, coma, stroke, death. The patient and his son understood the above complications and the procedure in detail and they agreed for the surgery.

OPERATIVE PROCEDURE: Patient was identified in the holding area appropriately and was brought to the operating room on a stretcher in a supine position. The patient was moved to the operating table and was intubated and general anesthesia was initiated. All the pressure points were padded well and the patient got of 2 grams of ANCEF preoperative antibiotic with intermittent stocking compression devices were applied to both lower extremities for DVT prophylaxis. The patient was positioned on a horseshoe head holder with the Mayfield frame and a small bump was placed under the right shoulder. Right side of the scalp hair was clipped and was prepped using ChloraPrep sponges and then ChloraPrep solution. The previous craniectomy incision was then identified and was draped in a sterile fashion. Timeout was performed as per the Main Line Hospital protocol.

Incision was done using a 10 number scalpel blade along the previous craniectomy incision. Using the monopolar cautery incision was carried down all the way to the bone. Using Gerald forceps and Metzenbaum scissors plane was created under the galea and over the duraplasty and a skin flap was elevated and was retracted forward. The craniectomy bone defect was exposed all around in the frontal, temporal and parietal regions. Bone flap was identified correctly and was soaked in the BETADINE solution for over 60 minutes. Next attention was paid to placing the mini plates and screws on the bone flap. Once the mini screws and plates were fixed on the bone flap it

Page 1 of 2

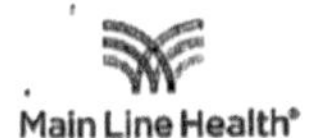

eOperative and Procedure Report - 5/31/2017 - 1 pg(s)

MAIN LINE HOSPITALS

Lankenau Hospital

OPERATIVE REPORT

Patient Name: RUDLOFF,STEPHEN
MR#: 765629

was brought into the operating field and was sized appropriately and was placed and used to cover the craniectomy defect. Bone flap was fixed in place by using the mini screws and plates. Bone flap was appropriately fitting. Thorough hemostasis was achieved with monopolar and bipolar cautery with a FloSeal and thrombin. Thorough irrigation with BACITRACIN solution and saline was done up to 3 liters. A 10-French flat JP drain was placed on the bone flap and was tunneled out with a separate incision. After achieving total hemostasis scalp flap was closed in layers using 2-0 Vicryl for galea layers and staples were used to close the skin. BACITRACIN ointment was applied and Telfa and 4 x 4 sponges were placed and a head wrap was applied. The drain was secured in place with a 3-0 nylon. The patient was extubated in the OR and was following commands and in a stable condition. He was transferred to ICU in a stable condition. All the counts of sponges and needles were correct at the end of the procedure. There were no complications encountered. No specimens were sent.

Ravichandra Madineni, MD

Dictated by:

DD: 06/07/2017 11:08:58
DT: 06/07/2017 11:49:59
427541/Dict Job #: 2257101
iChart Voice #: 63950900/iChart Text #: 57116229

CC: Ravichandra Madineni, MD,

Signed by Madineni, Ravichandra on 08-Jun-2017 11:07:02 -04:00

. Page 2 of 2 - Printed By:CUSTDM10\JOKF_stm_server On:12/13/2017 9:39:22 PM -05:00

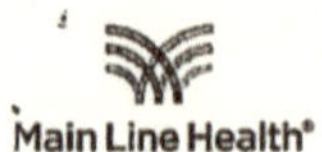

Main Line Health®

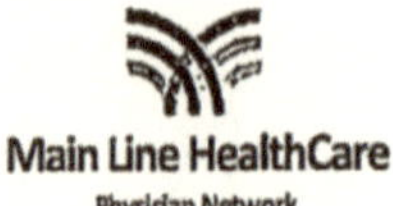

Main Line HealthCare

Physician Network

Main Line Healthcare Neurosurgery

Tel 610.525.1061
Fax 610.525.3509
mainlinehealth.org/mlhc

830 Old Lancaster Road
Medical Office Building North, Suite 209
Bryn Mawr, PA 19010

June 19, 2017

Anthony J. DeSalvo, D.O.
850 West Chester Pike
Suite 201
Havertown, PA 19083

Re: STEPHEN RUDLOFF
DOB: 10/22/1947

Dear Dr. DeSalvo:

Mr. Rudloff is here in the Neurosurgery Clinic for a followup from surgery that he had on May 31, 2017. The patient is about two week from cranioplasty on the right side that was done at Lankenau Hospital. The patient is doing well. He complains of having some soreness when he is chewing on the right temporal region, and complains of some pain along the incision. The patient denies having any headaches, nausea, vomiting, any seizures, or visual disturbances.

NEUROLOGICAL EXAMINATION: The patient is awake, alert, and oriented x3. Pupils are bilaterally round and reactive to light. Extraocular movements are intact. Visual field exam shows left-sided homonymous hemianopia. Strength is 5/5 in all extremities in all muscle groups. Sensation is normal to light touch and pinprick. The wound is completely healed. Staples were removed at this visit.

ASSESSMENT AND PLAN: I recommended that the patient get formal visual field evaluation done by ophthalmologist for evaluation of his driving ability. The patient is accompanied by his son at this visit, and I went over the plan of not doing any physical activity for four weeks. He is okay to do mild treadmill or stationary bike at the end of six weeks from surgery. Continue the Keppra which he is on for at least ninety days from surgery.

Please call our office with any further questions.

Sincerely,

ELECTRONICALLY SIGNED BY Ravi Chandra Madineni, MD ON 06/22/2017 13:12
Ravi Chandra Madineni, MD

cc: Anthony J. DeSalvo, D.O., 850 West Chester Pike, Suite 201, Havertown, PA 19083,
        FAX: 610-789-7836

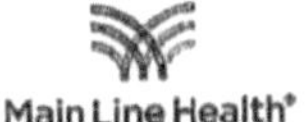

Main Line Health®

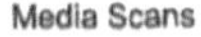

Main Line HealthCare

Physician Network

Main Line Healthcare Neurosurgery

Tel 610.525.1061
Fax 610.525.3509
mainlinehealth.org/mlhc

830 Old Lancaster Road
Medical Office Building North, Suite 209
Bryn Mawr, PA 19010

February 05, 2018

Anthony J. DeSalvo, D.O.
850 West Chester Pike
Suite 201
Havertown, PA 19083

Re: STEPHEN RUDLOFF
DOB: 10/22/1947

Dear Dr. DeSalvo:

CHIEF COMPLAINT: Right-sided cranioplasty flap resorption.

HISTORY OF PRESENT ILLNESS: Mr. Rudloff is a pleasant, 70-year-old gentleman who is well known to the Neurosurgery Service since he had a right-sided decompressive hemicraniectomy in February of 2017 for an intracerebral hemorrhage, and subsequently had a cranioplasty in June of 2017. The patient was routinely being evaluated with a CT scan of the head as well as CT angiogram for workup for a stroke, and was noticed to have resorption of the cranioplasty flap. The patient is here for followup for the same. The patient says he feels some numbness and tingling in the cranioplasty area along the incision line, and he also notices that he gets a sharp pain on and off when he feels there is more of abnormal sensation when he touches the scalp on the right side and also complains of a feeling of fullness or swelling on that side. No history of headache, nausea, or vomiting. No history of any weakness of the upper or lower extremities. No history of any fevers or any seizures.

NEUROLOGICAL EXAMINATION: Mr. Rudloff is a pleasant, 70-year-old gentleman who is awake, alert, and oriented x3. Pupils are equal and reactive to light. Extraocular movements are intact. Visual field exam shows a left-sided homonomous hemianopsia on confrontation test. Face is symmetric. Normal in strength. Tongue is midline. Strength is 5/5 in the upper and lower extremities in all muscle groups. Sensation is normal to light touch and pinprick. No redness or any discharge noticed along the incision line.

DATA REVIEW: CBC reveals a normal white count, as well as ESR and CRP are normal, and blood cultures are negative. CT scan of the head done on January 22, 2018 revealed partial resorption of the bone flap, most prominently in the posterior parietal region, as well as the temporal region with tinting of the remaining bone flap as well. No intracranial pathology noticed with evidence of a previous ICH and encephalomalacia of the right paraoccipital region.

ASSESSMENT AND PLAN: Mr. Rudloff is a 70-year-old gentleman who is about seven months after having cranioplasty of the right side, and now noticed to have resorption of the bone flap for which is a well known complication or natural progression after a bone flap placement with autologous bone. It has been well described in the literature with occurrence rate from 4% to 30%. Most of the time, this happens to be an aseptic resorption process; however, we cannot rule out an underlying, low-grade infection. I discussed the case with the Infectious Disease doctors, and I think at this point the patient needs to have removal of his

63

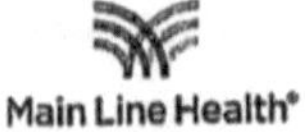

Main Line Health®

RUDLOFF, STEPHEN
February 05, 2018
Page 2

existing bone flap and replacement with a synthetic bone flap and cranioplasty. I explained the situation to the patient, as well as had a discussion with the patient's son over the phone. I think at this point I will consider giving him doxycycline 100 mg b.i.d. as a prophylactic for surgery, and will order the cranioplasty synthetic flap from Striker after reviewing the CT to fasten the bone flap. I expect the bone flap to be ready in about two to three weeks' time, and we will schedule him for surgery at that point. Doxycycline will be called in to the pharmacy, and the patient will be able to get the medication from there. The patient and the patient's son understand the treatment plan, and will call our office with any further questions.

Please call our office if you have any further questions.

Sincerely,

ELECTRONICALLY SIGNED BY Ravi Chandra Madineni, MD ON 02/12/2018 08:44
Ravi Chandra Madineni, MD

cc: Anthony J. DeSalvo, D.O., 850 West Chester Pike, Suite 201, Havertown, PA 19083,
        FAX: 610-789-7836

On September 17, 2020, I went to see Dr. Scharff in his office to have him look at the lump on the back of my neck. He checked it out and informed me it was a cyst. He informed me it was wide and deep. It had to come out. He set me up for preadmission tests at Lankenau Hospital on September 29, 2020. I got to the hospital on the twenty-ninth of September; the nurse took blood work, chest X-ray, EKG test, blood pressure, and oxygen level. The nurse gave me a coronavirus test. It came back negative, and the nurse informed me that the doctor had set up the operation for October 2, 2020. I was taken to the hospital on October 2 for the surgery by my neighbor, Alan. He dropped me off. I went into the hospital and checked in at 7:00 a.m. A nurse came out and took me back to get ready for the surgery. The doctors and nurses came in and put an IV on my arm. The doctor came in and informed me that he was going to give me local anesthesia. After the operation, I came back to my recovery room, and the doctor informed me that the surgery went well. I was all bandaged up with sutures. The doctor told me to keep the wound dry for two days; then, I could take a shower. The doctor informed me to call the office on Monday, October 5, to set up a follow-up appointment to check out my neck. The office had set me up to see Dr. Scarf on Wednesday, October 7, 2020. I went to see the doctor, and my wound was swollen. He put a needle in my neck and drained the fluid out. He put new bandages on a told me to go home and put ice on the area for twenty minutes. Every hour for twenty-four hours. He also informed me the cyst was benign. I was all done with the doctor. The doctor informed me that after forty eight hours if the swelling did not subside, call him.

As of October 9, 2020, the swelling went down on my neck by putting ice packs on the neck every twenty minutes, as suggested by the doctor. I feel fine now. I can go back to my normal routines now.

PROCEDURE: Right burr hole and evacuation of subdural hematoma

SURGEON: Robert Elliott, MD

ANESTHESIA: General endotracheal.

ESTIMATED BLOOD LOSS: 10 mL

SPECIMEN: None

COMPLICATIONS: None.

DRAIN: A 7-mm flat Jackson-Pratt drain.

FINDINGS: Xanthochromic CSF in epidural/subdural space under slight pressure

INDICATIONS FOR SURGERY:
The details of the patient's history, presentation, and examination are documented in detail
in my consultation note. I discussed the risks and rationale of surgery in detail with the
patient and family.

OPERATIVE PROCEDURE:

The patient was brought into the operating room. All lines and monitors were placed by the
anesthesia. The patient was induced with general anesthesia and intubated without
difficulty. A shoulder roll was placed under the right shoulder, and the head was turned to
the left exposing the right side of the scalp. Hair was shaved at the planned operative
sites (along the existing incision near vertex). Staples were removed. The scalp was
scrubbed, prepped and draped in usual sterile fashion. A total of 10 cc of 1% lidocaine
with epinephrine were injected into the planned incision sites.

I used a 10 blade to incise the scalp. Bipolar electrocautery was used to obtain hemostasis
and Bovie to perform a subperiosteal dissection exposing the outer table of the skull and
the PEEK plate. Self retaining retractors were placed. Throughout the case Ancef
irrigation was used. I used a drill to make a small burr hole through the PEEK plate and
immediately xanthochromic CSF under pressure came out from the epidural/subdural
space. I irrigated out this fluid.

An 11 blade was then used to make a stab incision just superior to the incision, and a
7-mm flat Jackson-Pratt drain was then tunneled subdural space and secured in place with
3-0 nylon sutures. It sas placed to minimal/thumbprint impression suction. The scalp was
then closed with inverted interrupted 2 -0 Vicryl sutures. The skin closed with interrupted
2-0 Ethibond sutures. Sterile dressing were then applied. All counts of needles, sponges,
Cottonoid, and instruments were correct. The patient was then transferred to the PACU in
stable clinical status.

Robert E. Elliott, MD

Case Information

✎ General Information

Date: **6/12/2021**   Time: **1600**   Status: **Posted**
Location: **LMC OR**   Room: **OR 01**   Service: **Neurosurgery**
Patient class: **Inpatient**   Case classification:

▣ Panel Information With CPT Code

Panel 1

Surgeon	Role	Procedure	Laterality	Anesthesia
Elliott, Robert E, MD	Primary	**Right sided burr hole and drainage of subdural/epidural collection [61312 (CPT®)]**	Right	General

Diagnosis Information

Diagnoses
History of cranioplasty

Brief Op Notes

No notes of this type exist for this encounter.

Op Notes

Op Note by Elliott, Robert E, MD at 6/12/2021 4:30 PM   Version 1 of 1

Author: **Elliott, Robert E, MD**   Service: **Neurosurgery**   Author Type: **Physician**
Filed: **6/12/2021 5:11 PM**   Date of Service: **6/12/2021 4:30 PM**   Status: **Signed**
Editor: Elliott, Robert E, MD (Physician)

OPERATIVE REPORT

PREOPERATIVE DIAGNOSES: 1) Subdural fluid collection after cranioplasty

POSTOPERATIVE DIAGNOSES: Same

Visualized paranasal sinuses and mastoid air cells: Mild bilateral ethmoidal mucosal thickening.

CT C spine and brain from 11/2/20:
1. No evidence of acute intracranial hemorrhage or calvarial fracture. Stable chronic findings as described above.
2. No acute fracture or dislocation is demonstrated throughout the cervical spine. There are multilevel discogenic and degenerative changes as described above.
3. Atheromatous calcification of the left carotid bifurcation.

Images were personally reviewed by myself and with the patient.

Assessment and Plan: In summary, Stephen J Rudloff is a 73 y.o. male who is s/p right ICH with evacuation, and cranioplasty in 2017 and subsequent right sided cranioplasty with synthetic bone on 3/14/2018 for bony reabsorption. Patient continues to have residual left-sided homonymous hemianopia. He developed clicking sensation with palpation on his skull about three weeks ago and suffered a fall this past November. The mini screws and plates loosened after this fall. He also started noticing small bumps on the scalp after the fall and which have been recurring with tenderness. He wished to proceed with the replacement of the cranial implant which was performed on 6/3/2021. He developed left upper extremity weakness as well as headache in the postoperative phase. He was found to have a subdural collection which was evacuated via bur hole on 6/12/2021. He is doing well postoperatively. Remaining sutures were removed at today's visit. I will see him back in 6 week's time. The patient expressed understanding, agrees with the overall plan and will follow up stated above. Thank you for giving opportunity to take care of Mr. Rudloff.

I, Abby Yochim PA-C, am scribing for, and in the presence of, Dr. Madineni,MD.

I, Dr. Ravi Chandra Madineni,MD personally performed the services described in this documentation as scribed by Abby Yochim PA-C in my presence, and it is accurate and complete.

Instructions

📅 Return in about 6 weeks (around 8/6/2021).

After Visit Summary (Printed 6/25/2021)

Additional Documentation

Vitals:	BP 124/80 Pulse 76 SpO2 94%
Flowsheets:	MLH Custom Formula Data
Encounter Info:	Billing Info, History, Allergies, Reviewed This Encounter

Communications

✉ Letter sent to Anthony J Desalvo, DO
   Sent 7/19/2021

Orders Placed

None

COMPLICATIONS: None.

ESTIMATED BLOOD LOSS: 50ml

DRAINS: None

INDICATION FOR PROCEDURE: Stephen J Rudloff is a 73 y.o.-year-old male who has a previous history of right-sided ICH undergoing decompressive craniectomy and subsequently cranioplasty with autologous bone which will be resolved so had synthetic flap cranioplasty between 2017 and 2018. Patient has been noticing significant discomfort and pain around the cranioplasty site with multiple fibrous nodules over the last 12 months . Extensive work-up with MRI and CT of the head did not reveal any pathology however there was loosening of the flap on palpation and pain on palpation around the anchor plates so plan was made for reexploration and removal of the existing cranial flap and replacement with a another synthetic cranial flap.

I discussed the procedure and as well as the complications in detail with patient .   Risks included, but not limited to, infection, bleeding, paralysis, seizures, stroke, weakness of the left side of the body, sensory dysfunction, CSF leak, need for further procedure, coma, stroke, death. The patient understood the above complications and the procedure in detail and agreed for the surgery.

NEED FOR ASSISTANT:
The first assistant was integral to the surgical case, assisting in the preparation and positioning of the patient, exposure and visualization of the operative field, retraction, irrigation and protection of key structures including the dura and cerebral cortex. Additionally, the first assistant prepared and plated the bone flap.   The assistant also helped in multi-layer closure and application of dressings. This assistance decreased risk of damage to neuronal structures, as well as decreased overall operative time, thereby decreasing risk of infection, overall anesthetic given to the patient , development of deep venous thrombosis and operative cost.

OPERATIVE PROCEDURE: Patient was identified in the holding area appropriately and was brought to the operating room on a stretcher in a supine position. The patient was moved to the operating table and was intubated and general anesthesia was initiated. All the pressure points were padded well and the patient received 2 g Ancef preoperative antibiotic with intermittent stocking compression devices were applied to both lower extremities for DVT prophylaxis. The patient was positioned on a horseshoe head holder with the Mayfield frame and a small bump was placed under the right shoulder. Right side of the scalp hair was clipped and was prepped using ChloraPrep sponges and then ChloraPrep solution. The previous craniectomy incision was then identified and was draped in a sterile fashion. Timeout was performed as per the Main Line Hospital protocol.

Incision was done using a 10 number scalpel blade along the previous craniectomy incision. Using the monopolar cautery incision was carried down all the way to the bone. Using Gerald forceps and Metzenbaum scissors plane was created under the galea and over the duraplasty and a skin flap was elevated and was retracted forward. After exposing the all anchor titanium mini plates around the cranial flap it was noticed that all the screws were loose and there was fibrous tissue that was growing around the mini plates. Anchoring mini screws and mini plates were removed and cranial flap was removed as well. Thorough irrigation with antibiotic saline was performed and a custom made synthetic cranial flap was placed and anchored with titanium mini plates and screws

IMPRESSION: Significant increase in size of the extra-axial collection along the right
frontoparietal convexity, with new mass effect and midline shift.
There is increased density within the collection, uncertain if this represents
blood products or due to an infectious process.

CT HEAD WITHOUT IV CONTRAST 6/3/21
IMPRESSION:
Postsurgical changes revision of the right cranioplasty. No acute intracranial abnormality.

CT of the head done on 3/2/2021:
COMPARISON: Head CT dated 11/2/2020.
--
IMPRESSION:
1. Unchanged appearance status post prior right parietotemporooccipital cranioplasty with
extensive cystic encephalomalacia in the subjacent parietal occipital convexity. There is no
overlying acute soft tissue abnormality.
2. No evidence of acute infarct, hemorrhage, mass or mass effect.

COMMENT:
Postoperative change: See impression.
Brain parenchyma: See impression.
Ventricles, cisterns, and sulci: Ex vacuo enlargement of the atrium and occipital horn of the
right lateral ventricle but otherwise normal in size and configuration.
Calvarium and extra cranial soft tissues: Otherwise unremarkable.
Visualized paranasal sinuses and mastoid air cells: Mild bilateral ethmoidal mucosal thickening.

CT C spine and brain from 11/2/20:
1. No evidence of acute intracranial hemorrhage or calvarial fracture. Stable chronic findings
as described above.
2. No acute fracture or dislocation is demonstrated throughout the cervical spine. There are
multilevel discogenic and degenerative changes as described above.
3. Atheromatous calcification of the left carotid bifurcation.

Images were personally reviewed by myself and with the patient.

Assessment and Plan: In summary, Stephen J Rudloff is a 73 y.o. male who is s/p right ICH
with evacuation, and cranioplasty in 2017 and subsequent right sided cranioplasty with
synthetic bone on 3/14/2018 for bony reabsorption. Patient continues to have residual left-
sided homonymous hemianopia. He developed clicking sensation with palpation on his
skull. about three weeks ago and suffered a fall this past November. The mini screws and
plates loosened after this fall. He also has started noticing small bumps on the scalp after the
fall and which have been recurring with tenderness. He wished to proceed with the
replacement of the cranial implant which was performed on 6/3/2021. He developed left upper
extremity weakness as well as headache in the postoperative phase. He was found to have a
subdural collection which was evacuated via bur hole on 6/12/2021. He is doing well
postoperatively. Staples were removed at today's visit. I will see him back in 1 week's time as
he still has sutures in place. The patient expressed understanding, agrees with the overall plan
and will follow up stated above. Thank you for giving opportunity to take care of Mr. Rudloff.

I, Abby Yochim PA-C, am scribing for, and in the presence of, Dr. Madineni,MD.

Case Information

✎ General Information

Date: **6/3/2021**
Location: **LMC OR**
Patient class: **Surgery Admit**

Time: **0700**
Room: **OR 10**
Case classification:

Status: **Posted**
Service: **Neurosurgery**

▣ Panel Information With CPT Code

Panel 1

Surgeon	Role	Procedure	Laterality	Anesthesia
Gomola, Ashley V, PA C	Assisting	**Right sided CRANIOPLASTY with removal of bone flap [62143 (CPT®)]**	**Right**	General
Madineni, Ravichandra, MD	Primary	REGULAR BED WITH MAYFIELD/HORSESHOE; STRYKER PEEK IMPLANT		

Diagnosis Information

Diagnoses
Skull defect

Brief Op Notes

Brief Op Note by Gomola, Ashley V, PA C at 6/3/2021 7:50 AM   Version 1 of 1

Author: **Gomola, Ashley V, PA C**
Filed: **6/3/2021 12:21 PM**

Service: **Neurosurgery**
Date of Service: **6/3/2021 7:50 AM**

Author Type: **Physician Assistant**
Status: **Signed**

Editor: Gomola, Ashley V, PA C (Physician Assistant)

Cosigner: Madineni, Ravichandra, MD at 6/3/2021 3:19 PM

Right sided CRANIOPLASTY with removal of bone flap (R) Procedure Note

Procedure: Right sided CRANIOPLASTY with removal of bone flap
CPT(R) Code: 62143 - PR REPLACE SKULL PLATE/FLAP

Pre-op Diagnosis
 * Skull defect [M95.2]

SCREW 1.5 X 4MM UNIII AXS SD - SN/A - LOG404405	Screw	SCREW 1.5 X 4MM UNIII AXS SD	N/A	STRYKER CRANIO	N/A	Right	12	Implanted

Complications: None; patient tolerated the procedure well.

Disposition: PACU - hemodynamically stable.

Condition: stable

Madineni, Ravichandra, MD
Phone Number: 610-525-1061

Op Notes

Op Note by Madineni, Ravichandra, MD at 6/3/2021 7:50 AM   Version 1 of 1

Author: Madineni, Ravichandra, MD   Service: Neurosurgery   Author Type: Physician

Filed: 6/19/2021 11:12 AM   Date of Service: 6/3/2021 7:50 AM   Status: Signed

Editor: Madineni, Ravichandra, MD (Physician)

OPERATIVE REPORT

Patient: Stephen J Rudloff
DOB: 10/22/1947

Date of Procedure: 6/3/2021

PREOPERATIVE DIAGNOSIS: Right sided cranial flap malfunction

POSTOPERATIVE DIAGNOSIS: Right-sided cranial flap malfunction

PROCEDURE: Right-sided removal of synthetic cranial flap and cranioplasty with PEEK cranial flap

SURGEON: Dr. Ravi Chandra Madineni MD

ASSISTANT: Ashley Gomola, PA-C

ANESTHESIA: General endotracheal.

SPECIMENS: Nil.

Last Chapter

On November 2, 2020, at 9:00 a.m., I left my apartment on Eagle Road and walked toward West Chester Pike in Havertown, Pennsylvania, to go to the bank. I crossed the street toward Ace Hardware Store. The traffic light was red, and the grass was high at that time. A piece of copper pipe was in the grass. I did not see the pipe. I tripped and fell on the sidewalk and hit the right side of my head on a section of black PVC pipe sticking out of the ground. I busted my right knee and my right hand wide open. I was bleeding pretty badly.

I was knocked out for a few moments. I got up and walked into the bank to get help. The people in the bank gave me paper towels for the bleeding. They informed me to go to the hospital. It did not look good. I left the bank and walked back home to my apartment.

I got a hold of my neighbor, and he took me to Bryn Mawr Hospital. I arrived at the hospital at 9:40 a.m. The nurses and doctors treated me. They took x-rays of my right hand and knee. I got a CAT scan and MRI tests. They gave me Tylenol. I got a CAT scan of the cervical spine also. Around 2:15 p.m., they released me from the hospital to go home. I got an Uber driver to pick me up and take me back to my apartment. I was informed by the nurses and doctors to get a follow-up with my primary doctor, Dr. Anthony De Salvo, in Havertown, Pennsylvania. I called Dr. De Salvo's office. He called me back to see how I was doing. We talked for a bit, and he informed me I have a follow-up with Dr. Margolies on November 23 at Lankenau

Hospital. I informed the doctor that I was having pain on the right side of my head, on the top of my head, my right knee, and my right hand. He gave me a script for physical therapy. I started physical therapy on the twenty-seventh of November 2020, three days a week for sixty days.

On February 15, 2021, I went to see my neurologist, Dr. Margolies; he gave me a complete physical. He saw the numerous lumps on the right side of my head. He informed me to go see Dr. Madineni, a neurosurgeon. He reviewed my script for physical therapy again for sixty more days, three times a week. On Monday, March 1, 2021, I went to see a neurosurgeon, Dr. Madineni, to show him all the lumps on the right side of my head. He gave me a complete physical exam. He went over all the problems I was having with pain in my head, my balance, and my eyesight again. The doctor informed me to go and get another CAT scan of my head. The next day, I set up the CAT scan of my head at Bryn Mawr Hospital. On March 4, 2021, Dr. Madineni called me to go see a skin cancer doctor, Dr. Mac Farlane, to see if she could use a cream or medication to dissolve the lumps on the right side of my head. Dr. Mac Farlane and Dr. Halgrin informed me that it was out of their hands. On April 23, 2021, they would fax a letter to Dr. Madineni that he would have to operate on me only. On April 30, 2021, I went to see Dr. Madineni, a neurosurgeon; we spoke about Dr. Mac Farlane's report. He informed me to get another MRI soft tissue test. On May 3, 2021, I went to Main Line Health Center in Broomall to get the MRI test. Dr. Madineni called me and informed me that they would have to remove the top of my head again because of the damage done from the fall I had on November 2.

On May 4, 2021, I went to see my primary doctor, Dr. De Salvo. He took blood work from me and sent a copy to the cardiologist, Dr. Kornberg. On May 5, I went in to see Dr. Kornberg at Lankenau Hospital for tests and a physical exam. He gave me an echocardiogram, chest x-rays, and EKG test. On May 14, I went to physical therapy for the last time and informed the therapist, Paul, that I would return when the doctors allowed me to go back to therapy, probably not until after Labor Day. On May 19, 2021, I went in to see Dr. Kornberg, a cardiologist, for a final checkup on the heart area. He informed me that he would send a copy to Dr. De Salvo, my primary doctor, that I was clear for surgery. On June 1, 2021, I went to Lankenau Hospital for preadmission to the hospital for numerous tests, bloodwork, EKG tests, and x-rays of the chest. The doctor came into the room, asked questions, and informed me, "You are good to go for surgery." On June 3, 2021, I was to report to the hospital at 5:30 a.m. On June 3, 2021, at 5:30 a.m., my son, Stephen, picked me up at my apartment and took me to Lankenau Hospital. He dropped me off at the front door. My son, Stephen, said goodbye to me and wished me good luck. He could not come into the hospital with me because of the coronavirus. I checked in at the hospital, and about one hour later, the nurse came into the waiting room and took me to the fourth-floor area. I got undressed and got onto the bed, and the nurses and doctors came in to get me ready for surgery.

They checked my vitals and asked questions. They gave me a double port IV on my right wrist. Dr. Madineni came in to talk with me. Then the anesthesia doctor and two nurses came into the room. They were to stay with me during the operation. The operation would be about four to five hours from start to finish. They took the top of my head off and removed the skull bone. I was sedated with morphine. Dr. Madineni came into the ICU to see me and informed me that everything went well. Both of my sons were notified by text. On June 4, my male nurse came into my room to see me. I pressed the button. I informed the nurse that my left wrist was black and blue. And I was in pain. He removed the arterial line from my wrist and put a pressure bandage on the area for a couple of days. On June 5, the house doctors came into my ICU and checked me out and informed me I was going to be discharged Sunday, June 6, at 1:00 p.m. My son, Edward, was informed. He picked me up at the front doors of the hospital. I got the discharge papers and left. The name of the operation was a cranioplasty revision. I was informed by the doctor to have a follow-up with my primary doctor, Dr. De Salvo.

On Friday, June 11, 2021, I went in to see my primary doctor at his office. He checked me out and checked my vitals. He saw all the staples on the top of my head and the right side of my head.

The staples were glued in place. I went home that day, and everything was fine; I informed the doctor my left wrist was still sore and black and blue. Around 4 p.m., I was eating my dinner, and I kept dropping my fork. My left arm and hand went paralyzed. I started to get numbness in my lips and face and pains on the right side of my head. I called Dr. Madineni's office; the doctor told me to get to the hospital right away. I was in the emergency room for about four to five hours. The doctors and nurses ordered a CAT scan and MRI tests. They checked my vitals, installed another IV in my arm again, and gave chest x-rays and EKG. I explained what was going on. Dr. Madineni was out of town at this time. Dr. Elliott came in to see me and told me he had to operate on me again. I had a subdural fluid collection after the operation I had. The operation would be three to four hours. I would be back in the ICU for a few more days. The doctor had to drill a hole in my head on the top and the back of my head to install a tube to release the fluid in the brain area. He painted the area that he worked on green, so Dr. Madineni could see the new staples. I was in the hospital until June 16, 2021. My son, Stephen, picked me up at the hospital front doors that day at 1:00 p.m. I got my discharge papers at 12:30 a.m.

On June 16, 2021, they informed me to meet Dr. Madineni at his office at Lankenau Hospital on June 18 to get half of the staples on the top of my head removed and the tube out of the back of my head. The staples had to stay in for at least ten days. The longer the staples stay in, the harder they are to get out. Dr. Madineni and Dr. Abby Yochin removed half of the staples on the top of my head and removed staples on the right side of my head. It was the most painful procedure I had done in my life. The doctors checked me out after taking the staples out. I have to go back on June 25 to get the rest of the staples out. I went to the office; the doctors removed all the rest of the staples and checked out my vitals. Dr. Madineni gave me a script to get another CAT scan of my head.

On Monday, June 28, I went to Main Line Health in Broomall to get the CAT scan for Dr. Madineni and take it to his office. He called me that day, and everything looked good. On June 29, Main Line Health called me to tell me a nurse would come to my apartment three times in the first week to check out my head and take my vitals. The traveling nurse came out two times on the second week, and she was finished that week for good. I had physical therapy and occupational therapy twice at my apartment, and both were finished. On August 6, 2021, I had a follow-up office visit with Dr. Madineni. He gave me a complete physical and checked my vitals. Everything at this time was good, no lumps on top of my head and no lumps on the right side of my head. All the lumps on my head are all gone now because of the fall I had on November 2, 2020. The doctor informed me to see him in ninety days, November 5, 2021.

On August 17, I had a follow-up office visit with Dr. Margolies, a neurologist; he checked me out, took my vitals, and said I could walk at Veterans Park in Broomall and I could go to the gym to exercise. I could ride a stationary bike and use the rowing machine and the walking track. No swimming right now until I see Dr. Madineni in November.

I wore a bandana on my head for three weeks after the operation. I am still trying to get my balance back and my eyesight back again; it will take at least one to two years for the nerves to join together again.

Again, I want to thank Dr. Madineni, Abby, and the staff at both offices for all of their help and guidance with all of my surgeries. They told me that I have a good sense of humor, and I have a high tolerance for pain. I want to thank everybody who purchased this book. I hope you enjoyed it. Like I said at the beginning of this book, some of the proceeds from the sales of this book will go to Tunnel to Towers and Shriners Hospital for curing cancer in kids. I live my life like navy seals; no easy day than yesterday. I am a cancer survivor and a stroke survivor—brain bleed.

God bless all of you!

Dr. Madineni, thank you for saving my life again.

The End

About the Author

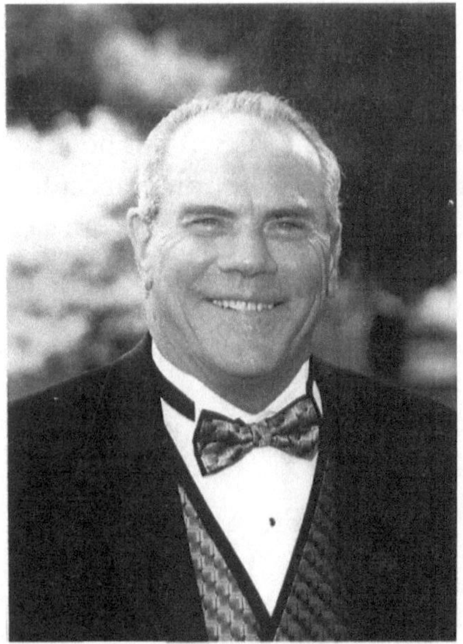

My name is Steve. I live in Havertown, Pennsylvania. I am a Vietnam War veteran. I was in the navy from 1966 to 1972. I hope you enjoy this book.

I wanted to tell this story because I realized that life is too short, and I wanted to give back to people who are worse off than me.

All the chapter in this book is fact-checked. And I tried to the best of my ability to give you all facts about my medical history.